Understanding Patients' Sexual Problems

A Reference Handbook for Healthcare Professionals

Grace Blodgett PhD MSN

To Hannah,
I wish you continued sexual happiness.
Dr. Gracie
November 27th, 2015

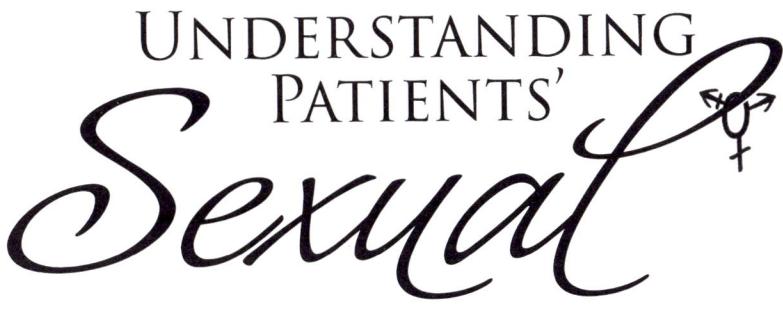

AVIVA PUBLISHING
New York

Understanding Patients' Sexual Problems
A Reference Handbook for Healthcare Professionals

Copyright @ 2015 by Grace Blodgett.

All rights reserved. No part of this publication may be reproduced, stored in a retrieval system, or transmitted in any form or by any means, electronic, mechanical, photocopying, recording, scanning, or otherwise, without the prior written permission of the author. Address all inquiries to:

Grace Blodgett
sexualitywithgrace@gmail.com
www.UnderstandingPatientsSexualProblems

ISBN: 9781940984704
Library of Congress #2015933547

Editor: Tyler Tichelaar
Jacket Design: Nicole Gabriel / www.AngelDogProductions.com
Interior Book Design: Nicole Gabriel / www.AngelDogProductions.com

Every attempt has been made to source properly all quotes. The author and publisher are not responsible for the accuracy of information on URLs included in this book. The Internet is always changing, but all quotes and URLs referenced in this book were current at the time of its publication.

Printed in United States of America

First Edition

10 9 8 7 6 5 4 3 2 1

To Peter, my husband, my love, and my best friend of 40 years.
To Mark, Paul, Kate, and Jonathan, our children;
and
To Gillian, Avery, Maysea, India, Isabelle, and Lilly, our granddaughters.
I love you all dearly.

In memory of Gloria, my dear friend of 55 years, who died August 14th, 2014

CONTENTS

Preface — 11
Organization of This Handbook — 13
Introduction — 19

SECTION 1 **SEXUALITY OF PEOPLE IN THE HEALTHCARE ENVIRONMENT**

Chapter 1 **Misconceptions and Misperceptions that Often Result in Miscommunication** — 25

Nurses' Sexuality
Physicians' Sexuality
Patients' Sexuality

SECTION 2 **SEXUAL BEHAVIORS AND SOCIAL FACTORS THAT INFLUENCE SEXUALITY IN AMERICA**

Chapter 2 **Sexual Behaviors and Techniques According to a Person's Sexual Orientation** — 43

Sexual Attraction and Sexual Orientation

Sexual Behaviors and Sexual Orientation

Lifestyles Based on Sexual Orientation

Chapter 3 **The Sexual Proclivities of American Adults, Societal Mores, and the Mass Media's Impact on Sexual Behavior** — 51

Sexual Dreams and Nocturnal Emissions
Sexual Fantasy
Flirting
Romantic and Limerent Love
Masturbation
Pornography
Prostitution
Sexual Scripting

SECTION 3   **SEXUAL BEHAVIOR PROBLEMS OF AMERICAN CHILDREN AND ADOLESCENTS**

Chapter 4   *Differentiating Between Expected Childhood Curiosity and Unexpected Sexual Behavior Problems of Children*   77

The Sexualization of American Girls

Gender Dysphoria in Children

Sexual Development Incongruence Due to a Chromosome Variance to include Turner Syndrome, Klinefelter Syndrome, XYY Syndrome, and Triple XXX Syndrome

Sexual Development Incongruence Due to a Hormonal Variance, to include Complete Androgen Insensitivity, Partial Androgen Insensitivity, and Mild Androgen Insensitivity

Hypospadias

Cryptorchidism (Undescended Testes)

Congenital Adrenal Hyperplasia

Child Sexual Abuse

Sexual Behavior Problems in Children

Female Genital Cutting

Sexually Transmitted Infections in Children

Chapter 5 **High Risk Sexual Behaviors By and Against Adolescents and the Challenges These Behaviors Present**   167

Sexual Coercion of Adolescents

Unintended Pregnancies in American Adolescents

Sexually Transmitted Infections in American Adolescents

Rape in American Adolescents

SECTION 4 **SEXUAL ISSUES THAT MAY RESULT FROM SEXUAL ORIENTATION, GENDER IDENTITY DYSPHORIA, AND/OR SEXUAL DEVELOPMENTAL VARIANCES**

Chapter 6 **Problems that Adults and Adolescents who are Gay, Lesbian, or Bisexual Experience as a Result of Their Sexual Orientation**   203

Problems Specific to Gay Youth, Adult Gay Males, and Bisexual Males
Problems Specific to Adolescent and Adult Lesbians and Bisexual Women

Chapter 7 **Sexual and Social Problems that Adults and Adolescents with Gender Dysphoria Encounter**   221

Personal Distress with Expressed and Experienced Gender and Secondary Sex Characteristics

Discrimination, Harassment, Transphobia

Fully Reversible, Partially Reversible, and Irreversible Interventions

Real-Life Experience (RLE)

SECTION 5 **STANDARD ADULT SEXUAL BEHAVIORS AND THEIR ASSOCIATED SEXUAL DYSFUNCTIONS**

Chapter 8 **Sexual Dysfunctions in Men and Women and the Learned Behaviors That Contribute to Those Dysfunctions**   237

Learned Behaviors

Low Sexual Desire Disorders in Men and Women

Erectile Disorder in Men and Lubrication Disorder in Women

Orgasm Disorders in Men and Women

Premature, Absent, and Retrograde Ejaculation Disorders in Men

Sexual Pain Disorders in Men (Dyspareunia) and Women (Vulvodynia)

Chapter 9 **Sexuality Concerns in Adults that Occur as a Result of a Chronic Illness, a Severe Disability, an End-of-Life Illness or Older Age**   299

Alzheimer's Disease and Sexuality

Cancer and Sexuality

Diabetes Mellitus and Sexuality
Multiple Sclerosis and Sexuality

Intellectual, Developmental, and Physical Disabilities and Sexuality

Older Individuals and Sexuality

Chapter 10 **High Sexual Desire Disorders and Sexual Compulsivity in Men and Women, and the Learned Behaviors that Contribute to Their Sexually Compulsive Actions** 353

Escalating Frequency and Intensity of Sexual Behaviors Significantly Impair or Prevent Emotional, Affectionate, Bonding Relationships

Behaviors Identified as Addictive, Obsessive Compulsive, High Sexual Desire or an Impulse Control Disorder

SECTION 6 **DSM-5 IDENTIFIED PARAPHILIAS AND PARAPHILIC DISORDERS, DSM-5 SPECIFIED AND UNSPECIFIED PARAPHILIC DISORDERS AND OTHER PARAPHILIC DISORDERS**

Chapter 11 **A General Overview of Paraphilias and Paraphilic Disorders. Eight DSM-5 Selected Paraphilias and Paraphilic Disorders, DSM-5 Specified and Unspecified Paraphilias and Paraphilic Disorders, and Examples of Non-DSM-5 Paraphilic Disorders** 365

General Overview of Paraphilias and Paraphilic Disorders

Eight DSM-5 Identified Paraphilias and Paraphilic Disorders, to include Exhibitionism Disorder, Fetishistic Disorder, Frotteuristic Disorder, Pedophilic Disorder, Sexual Sadism Disorder, Sexual Masochism Disorder, Transvestic Fetishism Disorder, Voyeuristic Disorder

DSM-5 Specified and Unspecified Paraphilic Disorders

Other Paraphilias and Paraphilic Disorders

Appendices — 421

Appendix A:	How Comfortable Are You with Your Own Sexuality?	423
Appendix B:	How Comfortable Are You with Patient Sexuality?	425
Appendix C:	Standard Sexual Assessment	427
Appendix D:	Examples of Therapies and Techniques Applied to Sexual Issues	429
Appendix E:	The Plissit Model of Sex Therapy	437
Appendix F:	Your Attitudes Toward Unconventional Sexual Behaviors	439
Appendix G:	Supportive Interventions Guide for Children	441
Appendix H:	Supportive Interventions Guide for Adults	445
Appendix I:	How Comfortable Are You with Childhood Sexuality?	447

References — 451
About the Author — 489

PREFACE

*"Do you not know how uncontrolled and
unreliable the average human being
is in all that concerns sexual life."*

— Sigmund Freud

Healthcare professionals (HCPs) demonstrate varying levels of knowledge, understanding, experience, and perceptions about the topic of sexuality in the patient care arena. Unfortunately, a great deal of the information about sexuality they bring to the clinical arena is often full of misconceptions and insecurities about their own sexuality, as well as that of the patients for whom they provide care. The contributing factors to these misconceptions and insecurities are the result of behaviors learned since early childhood, as well as a paucity of education about sexuality. Both can be unlearned and corrected.

Anecdotal comments and requests for assistance received over the past forty-plus years from HCPs from many areas of clinical practice clearly indicate that many HCPs feel helpless in a situation over which they feel they have little control. They have frequently expressed their concerns, discomfort, embarrassment, lack of confidence, and lack of knowledge. Sexuality is one of the remaining taboos in American society—a topic best avoided by HCPs for the sake of all involved.

I initially decided to write this manual to address the immediate and specific needs of nurses and nurse practitioners in many fields of healthcare as they applied to patient sexuality. The realization soon came that many HCPs, as well as nurses, experience similar concerns, anxieties, and questions about patient sexuality; consequently, this reference guide addresses the needs of all HCPs who provide direct patient care.

This handbook is not intended to be a complete medical textbook about human sexuality. Readers may use it as a reference book to turn to for answers to resolve patient sexual problems on an as needed basis, then seek further information from a full medical text.

ORGANIZATION OF THIS HANDBOOK

This handbook is a reference for researching specific sexual conditions and situations; topics can be read and researched out of sequence, rapidly, efficiently, and effectively. Information is presented in a way that is easy to use and so content retention and recollection are facilitated. It stands apart from most reference books of this nature because:

- It contains less narrative text, with more condensed information, lists, and bullet points than most textbooks.
- As many references as possible contain Internet addresses to facilitate retrieval of source materials.
- More attention and detailed information is given to topics that many HCPs find either 1) very difficult to manage or painful to confront, such as variances of sex development and child sexual abuse, or 2) are a major public health issue, such as sexually transmitted infections (STIs).

- It contains a number of questionnaires for completion by readers, the written responses to which are *for their eyes only*. Completion of these questionnaires may encourage HCPs to acknowledge certain aspects of their own sexuality that they may not have previously recognized. HCPs may also consider patients' sexuality issues more promptly and in greater depth.
- Distributed throughout this book are questions, topics for discussion, and quotations pertaining to the actual topic at hand that provide further insight into the discussion.
- Five sections and eleven chapters identify and describe both the conventional and non-conventional sexual behaviors and problems of Americans that occur both frequently and infrequently. Descriptions of interventions by HCPs for resolution of these sexual behaviors and problems follow immediately after their identification.
- All descriptions of sexual problems or conditions have the same format and the same headings to facilitate a faster read and increased retention, as well as contribute to successful implementation of interventions. These headings are: *Definition, Signs and Symptoms, Origins, Background, Therapeutic Interventions, Supportive Interventions,* and *Potential Outcomes*.

Section 1: Sexuality of People in the Healthcare Environment
Chapter 1 describes the sexuality of healthcare professionals

Organization of This Handbook

(HCPs), patients, and the public, and the perceptions that members of both groups have about themselves and about each other. This chapter is intended to increase HCPs' awareness of the dilemmas that all individuals in healthcare face when they first begin their interactive relationships and as those relationships progress toward resolution and completion.

Section 2: Sexual Behaviors and Social Factors that Influence Sexuality in America

Chapters 2 and 3 describe many of the conventional and non-conventional sexual behaviors of Americans, as well as the many social influences on sexuality that exist in America. Some have a positive influence on society; others do not.

Section 3: Sexual Behavior Problems of American Children and Adolescents

Chapters 4 and 5 address the sexual behaviors of children and adolescents that are considered to be normal and expected and result from childhood curiosity and inquisitiveness. They also describe the sexual behaviors of American children and adolescents that are problematic. Some topics in these chapters are described in greater detail than others, either due to the gravity of the conditions and the challenges presented or the increased frequency of occurrence.

Section 4: Sexual Issues that May Result from Sexual Orientation, Gender Identity Dysphoria, and/or Sex Developmental Variances

Chapter 6 contains the less-frequently encountered non-conventional, gay, lesbian, and bisexual sexual orientation behaviors of American adults. These sexual orientation-associated activities are considered lawful and are almost always acceptable to the involved individuals. However, they are not always accepted socially, and they are still considered to be non-conventional by many. The sexual problems directly associated with a gay, lesbian, or bisexual orientation are also found in this chapter.

Chapter 7 presents the sexual and social problems that occur in people with gender identity dysphoria (GD), together with the many associated problems that may occur as a result of adverse societal opinions.

Section 5: Standard Adult Sexual Behaviors and Their Associated Sexual Dysfunctions

Chapter 8 addresses many of the most frequently encountered *conventional* or *standard* sexual activities of American adults. These sexual behaviors are almost always considered lawful, accepted socially, and acceptable to the individual involved. Associated sexual dysfunctions that occur are also in this chapter.

Chapter 9 discusses sexuality concerns in adults that occur as a result of chronic illness, severe disability, an end-of-life illness or older age.

Chapter 10 presents the condition known as *s*exual hyperactivity or compulsivity (also referred to by some as sexual addiction), as well as non-paraphilic sexual disorders, and their effect on persons with this condition.

Section 6: DSM-5 Identified Paraphilias and Paraphilic Disorders, DSM-5 Specified and Unspecified Paraphilic Disorders and Other Paraphilic Disorders

Chapter 11 presents a complex topic, that of the sexual paraphilias and paraphilic disorders: sexual behaviors that are mostly against the law, unacceptable socially, and often unacceptable to the involved individual(s). This section contains descriptions of sexual practices that may be vastly different to those of the reader, so some may find them difficult to understand and accept. This makes the provision of unbiased, non-judgmental care for these individuals difficult at best.

Mark Twain once said: "*Like the moon, every one of us has a dark side.*" The paraphilias represent the dark side of American sexuality.

INTRODUCTION

"Throughout the history of nursing sexuality has been ignored both in relation to patient care and to nurses themselves, and the reasons lie deep in our culture."

— B.T. Basavanthappa

To be acknowledged as a profession, healthcare professionals (HCPs) have developed written standards for a member's expected performance within a particular profession or discipline. This specific body of written knowledge applies only to that membership, as well as compliance levels to which members are also expected to adhere. Many of these performance standards for HCPs include standards of performance and compliance that address and evaluate care as it applies to sexuality. Very few HCPs demonstrate that they meet their established standards as they apply to patient sexuality.

For example, nurses have worked hard over the past 50 years for the discipline of nursing to establish itself as a profession, and progress has been made toward achievement of that goal. The American Nurses Association (ANA), a representative body that developed the standards by which the discipline of nursing is measured, found that most nurses have complied with and achieved all of their standards *except* the standard of sexuality. Unfortunately, when it comes to compliance and completion of the 16 care standards as applied to sexual care, nurses show a less than stellar performance. The most frequent reasons cited by nurses for noncompliance are attributed to the anxiety that these discussions evoke as a result of inadequate sexual knowledge and preparation, and the incorrect assumption and declaration by members of the nursing profession that they just cannot talk with patients about sexuality.

Similarly, the discipline of medicine is clearly established as a profession through its standards of practice. The medical profession has its body of knowledge and expected levels for performance and compliance—almost everyone knows the physician's role. However, this does not mean that all physicians regularly adhere

Introduction

to those standards, and as with nurses, the standard they do not meet is that of management of patients' sexual needs. Like nurses, physicians feel it is not their job, and provide similar reasons for their non-compliance to their rules and expectations.

HCPs in general avoid the patients' sexual concerns, and they do their utmost to prevent any discomfort or confrontation. Instead, they move on to safer, more manageable situations in which they feel more confident in their knowledge, clinical skills, and abilities. This avoidance is not a malicious or conscious act; it happens as a result of their personal sexual insecurities and a lack of sexual knowledge, time, and confidence in their counseling skills. After 50 years as a registered nurse at most levels of practice, and 20 years in the sexology arena, I have seen and experienced many occasions when HCPs have floundered and searched for the right words and information they needed. HCPs have demonstrated a need for this information.

In this handbook, sexual behavior overall is described as well as attitudes toward sexuality that exist in America today. What its citizens actually do sexually as opposed to what the laws of the land say they should do are worlds apart, and perhaps they need to become more closely aligned. The sexual behaviors of different age groups are outlined, together with the presenting expressions of those behaviors. The self-identification and self-examination by HCPs of their sexual inhibitions, misconceptions, insecurities, and fears need to take place not only for their sexual health but for their patients' welfare.

This handbook's goals are threefold: 1) to encourage self-reflection by readers of their attitudes toward sexuality, 2) to promote the future inclusion of adequate information about patient sexuality in all HCP preliminary and continuing education curricula, and 3) to encourage HCPs to acknowledge and embrace patient sexuality and sexual problems with the same level of professionalism and confidence as they approach the patients' other healthcare needs.

SECTION 1

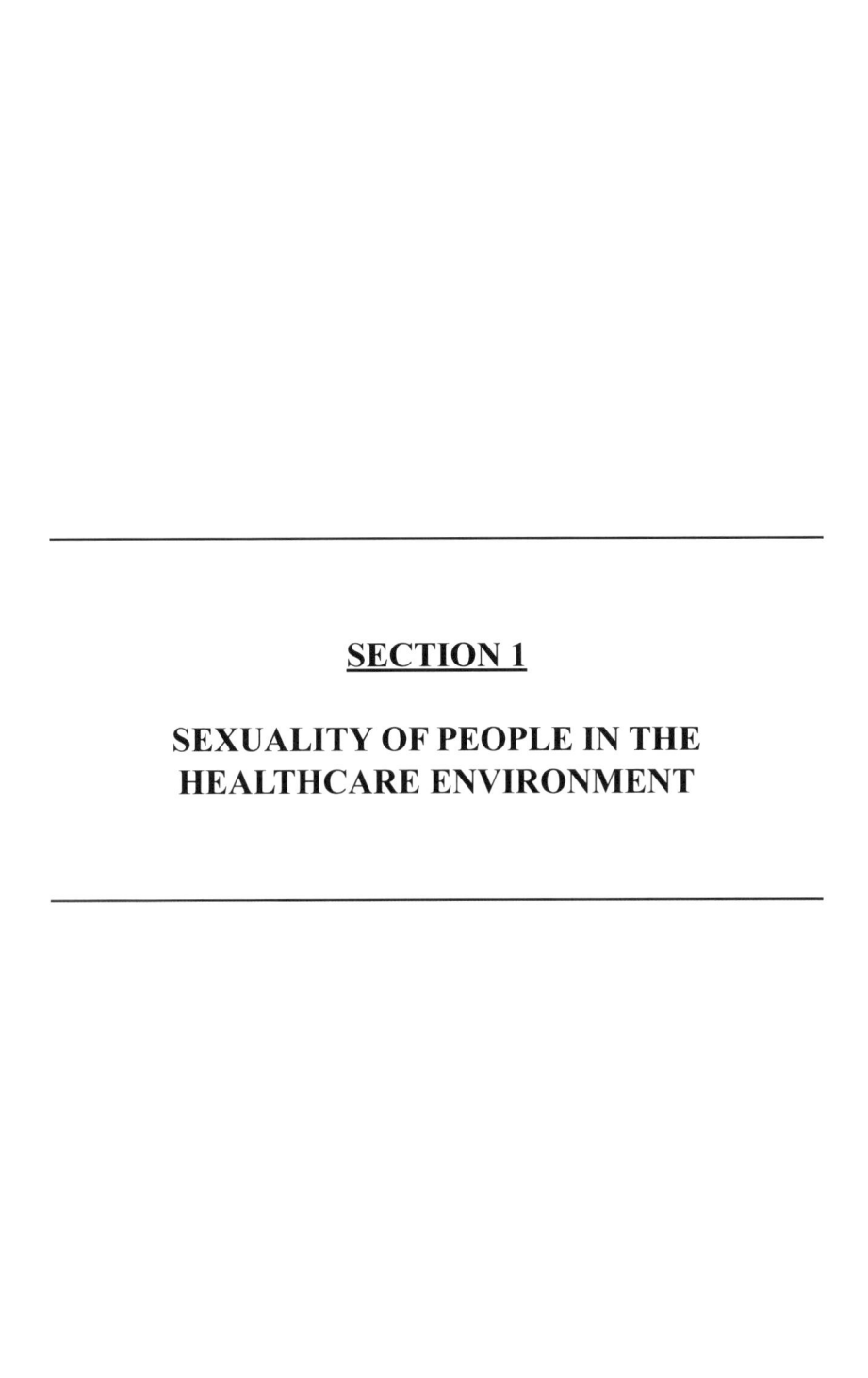

SEXUALITY OF PEOPLE IN THE HEALTHCARE ENVIRONMENT

CHAPTER ONE

MISCONCEPTIONS AND MISPERCEPTIONS THAT OFTEN RESULT IN MISCOMMUNICATION

"Sex lies at the root of life, and we can never reverence life until we know how to understand sex."

— Havelock Ellis

The healthcare environment that exists in America today is such that honest, direct, and healthy discussions between healthcare professionals and patients about patient sexuality issues are extremely difficult at best. This difficulty is the result of social beliefs that a person's sexuality is a private issue as well as the lack of education among healthcare professionals about sexuality and how to discuss it with patients. These difficulties also persist as the result of hundreds of years of history, culture, religion, and even turmoil that continue to influence all aspects of healthcare management and the practice of healthcare. A review of some of the conditions that lead to these differences are described below, according to the groups of people involved.

A. The sexualization of female nurses by themselves, patients, and the general public, and the perceptions held of them by patients and the general public

   1. The sexualization of nurses from their perspective
   - The majority of nurses are female (currently at approximately 90%), and the majority of research done on this topic has been performed on female nurses
   - Just as there are different opinions within the general public about what is natural and healthy about sex, different opinions exist among nurses. Nurses are fraught with the same insecurities about their sexual behavior, and have similar issues with regards to their attitudes toward sexuality and sexual behaviors, as other members of the public
   - The social mores, race, culture, place, politics, religion, etc. (social scripts) in which they were raised all influence nurses. In the area of sexuality, people are more influenced by those people with whom they had the greatest interaction as young children, specifically

their parents (parental scripts) or other first caregivers and family
- If children only learn negative scripts, they become adults whose sexual education may be limited. If their education is based on sexual myths and full of negative stereotypes, it may hinder their perceptions of others and themselves; children who become nurses are no exception (see Appendix A)
- A commonly held belief is that only a heterosexual relationship within the bond of marriage is an acceptable and healthy sexual relationship. While another belief, at the other end of the spectrum, is that *any* sexual activity that is consensual and does not invade the rights of others is acceptable and healthy. Like many others, nurses are scattered along the spectrum in their sexual beliefs
- Nurses assume their own position on the gender continuum, and difficulties arise for them when they either align themselves with or act in conflict with others along that continuum
- Nurses also potentially carry their sexual concerns or issues with them, which can hinder their ability to discuss sexuality openly and warmly with others
- When nurses hear untrue opinions and unkind names and statements expressed against them by some members of the public, they begin to internalize them.

Those statements may even become their actual beliefs about themselves
- Reynolds and Magnan [1(abstract)] found that nurses believe it is their role to meet the sexual concerns of the patient; however, "discomfort, embarrassment, or strongly held attitudes about the nurses' role in discussing sexuality with patients can act as barriers to these patient concerns." They also found that "Time availability and confidence in one's ability to address issues related to human sexuality present significant barriers to incorporating sexuality assessment and counseling into nursing practice"[1]
- Waterhouse[2(p412-418)] found that nurses acknowledge it is their professional responsibility to address patients' sexual issues, but they are not comfortable doing so
- Personal anecdotal comments received from nurses as to why they do not discuss sexuality with patients indicates the level of resistance that exists in the practice arena. Nurses claim they are too embarrassed, they were never taught how in nursing school, and such concerns are not a priority; they know hardly anything about the range of human sexuality themselves, let alone are able to teach others; they are too tongue-tied, and they don't want to offend the patient. "I know I should, but I can't, so I avoid it."

- Numerous papers contain various reasons nurses have given as to why they do not include sexuality within their nursing practice[3(p54)]

2. **The sexualization of nurses from the patients' perspective**
   - Both participants in the patient-nurse relationship bring their own sexual experiences and beliefs to the situation, but nurses bring an additional burden with them that adversely influences their delivery of quality nursing care—that of being a sexual stereotype
   - The images or stereotypes of nurses held by some members of the general public have changed frequently and dramatically, sometimes positively, sometimes negatively, from ancient times to the present. Nursing is perceived and portrayed as "being a metaphor for sex"[3(p54)]
   - Much of the blame for these negative images has been assigned to the media; however, the past thirty years have demonstrated that this issue is more complicated than just media involvement and blame. These endless references to the sexuality of nurses damages their reputation, the value and worth of the work they perform, and discounts their preparatory and continuing preparation, their hard work, and the commitment it takes to become a professional nurse

- Some names and descriptions used by the public for nurses are related to the historical religious and military roles of nurses, as well as nursing initially being a *calling* for women. These names and descriptions include: *angels in white, sweet, battleaxes, torturers, saintly domestics, bimbos, kind, drunken sots, witches in white, fannies, oversexed, handmaidens to physicians, unselfish and dedicated, Nurse Ratcheds, sexual playthings, and naughty night nurses*
- Why these derogatory terms are applied to nurses and why the profession of nursing has been selected as a target out of the female professions that exist (librarians, physical therapists, teachers, occupational therapists, etc.) is unclear
- Kalisch and Kalisch[4(p179-195)] examined the character depictions of 677 nurses and 466 doctors in films, television, and novels between 1920 and 1980. They found that there was a steady decline in the way nurses were depicted, while depictions of the doctors remained consistently positive or actually showed improvement. Female nurses were perceived as being "promiscuous playthings" for the physician and the patient, an "easy sexual harassment target; sexually provocative, and all-knowing about things sexual"
- Nurse researchers in England and Ireland recently

viewed the ten most-watched videos within 300,900 YouTube hits that showed a negative or positive image of nursing.[5] They examined them for language, actions, content, and intent, and the results classified nurses into three categories: *knower/doer, sexual plaything, and witless incompetent*

- Nurses are neither saints nor sinners; they have an important job to do and want to do it professionally and expertly without having inappropriate and denigrating names attached to them
- Nurses are encouraged to respond with thoughtful, proactive actions to stem this almost unending onslaught of offensive name calling. Accurate, honest, and responsible self-descriptions must be given by nurses of who they are and what they represent—intelligent, educated, skilled, knowledgeable professionals who fulfill one of society's absolutely essential roles, that of caring for the sick

B. The perceptions of physicians' sexuality, demeanor, and attitude, as seen by healthcare professionals, patients, and the general public

Less has been written or said about physicians' (generally male) sexuality than about the sexuality of nurses (generally female), possibly because physicians have always been seen in positions of power and perhaps not viewed as such an easy target to be sexualized by the media. For many years, medical doctors (MDs) have been revered by the public for their knowledge, skills, power, and charisma, as well as inspired awe in their role as *Captain of the Ship* for the healthcare team. As a result, MDs have often been seen to be full of intrigue and quietly unattainable by female patients and nurses alike, making them sexually attractive to both.

Thirty or so years ago marked the appearance of Health Maintenance Organizations (HMOs) and Preferred Provider Organizations (PPOs) in the management of the financial aspects in the healthcare arena, and consequently, delivery and management of patient care. The physician to all intents and purposes lost his leadership and power role as well as his elevated status within the community. Physicians in general have lost favor with the public and have "fallen from the pedestal." Patients, staff, and the public now often claim that physicians have been rude to patients, families, and staff; they lack public relations skills; they have temper tantrums; and overall, they show disruptive behavior within the healthcare setting. Unfortunately, most healthcare administrators have not managed these physicians and their unacceptable behaviors, primarily because physicians, especially surgeons, have always been the revenue-generators for hospitals, and as such, were beyond reprimand.

However, the past few decades have brought many changes within the healthcare arena to the extent that physicians are now expected to be contributing team members who treat other team members with respect and courtesy. Unfortunately, some physicians have not accepted this approach, and sexual harassment and verbal abuse by physicians of patients, relatives, residents, interns, medical students, and junior doctors continues. In some instances, harassment of doctors by other doctors has become yet another issue for healthcare administrators to manage.

1. **The Sexual Behavior of Some Male Physicians**
   Definition of Physician Sexual Harassment: Behavior that exploits patients and healthcare staff in a sexual way; it can be verbal or physical. "There are primarily two types of sexual misconduct: sexual impropriety and sexual violation. Both types are the basis for disciplinary action by the State Medical Board if the board determines that the behavior exploited the physician-patient relationship."[6(p1)]

   - Female physicians represent approximately 30% of the physician population
   - "Sexual impropriety may comprise the behavior, gestures, or expressions that are seductive, usually

suggestive, disrespectful of patient privacy, or sexually demeaning to a patient"[1]
- "Sexual violation may include physical contact between a physician and a patient, whether or not initiated by the patient, and engaging in any conduct with a patient that is sexual or may be construed as sexual...." [1(p2)]
- Sexual harassment of a patient by a physician signals the end of patient trust of the physician
- Physicians who sexually harass patients destroy the usual therapeutic patient-physician relationship necessary for optimal patient healing
- The professional working relationship between a physician and other HCPs adversely impacts when physicians sexually harass staff, and it often results in a hostile work environment
- Like it or not, physicians are held to a higher standard than others mainly because of the intimacy of the physician-patient relationship as well as the positions of relative wealth and status they maintain within the public arena
- Sexual harassment of patients by male physicians appears to have tainted the public's perception of the medical community as a whole

2. **Male Physicians as Victims of Sexual Harassment**
   - Although some of the allure associated with male

Misconceptions and Misperceptions

   physicians may have worn off, much remains, and some female patients are still attracted to them as persons of interest sexually, as well as financially
- In a survey by Haaretz[7] of 502 male physicians and 589 female physicians in 43 specialties in Israel, approximately 100 male respondents reported sexual harassment, with 46% of them saying that female patients were the perpetrators. Then 29% were by female colleagues, then 21% by female doctors in other departments, and 17% by female relatives
- Male and female senior colleagues sexually harassed just over one-quarter of the male respondents. Note: over 100% was achieved since more than one answer was possible

3. **Female Physicians as Victims of Sexual Harassment**
   - Less has been said about the sexuality of female physicians than nurses; however, as females, they also bear the brunt of sexual harassment, both by their male and female peers and male and female patients
   - Nearly half of the female physicians in the survey mentioned above had been sexually harassed at work, either physically or verbally, and of these, "60% said the culprit was a senior colleague."[7] Thirty-four percent of respondents said that the perpetrators "were colleagues in their own department[7(p1)]," and 26% colleagues in

other departments[7]
- Only recently have junior physicians begun to report their senior colleagues for sexual harassment; this might also be an indication of how senior physicians have lost some of their power over female junior physicians[7]
- Non-reporting by subordinates remains an issue because physicians have been known to terminate, withhold a raise or promotion, deny scholarships, fail students, etc.
- In a Canadian survey of 599 female physicians, more than 75% of respondents reported some sexual harassment by patients[8]

C. Interactions between patients and non-nurse/non-physician healthcare professionals are different to those between patients, nurses, and physicians

Very little research has evaluated the sexuality and impact of non-nurse healthcare professionals, such as pharmacists, physical therapists, dieticians, respiratory therapists, and occupational therapists. A frequently asked question is: Why are these other primarily female disciplines within the healthcare environment not sexualized to the extent of nurses?

- Potential answers to this question are:
  - Nurses perform intimate bodily care for patients who are virtual strangers without sexual implications or hesitation
  - Some believe that nurses might encourage or even welcome the sexual advances of others without resistance
  - Male patients perceive a loss of control of many aspects of their manhood when they enter the healthcare environment. They attempt to reclaim that loss of control by demeaning nurses either verbally through covert sexual innuendos and/or overt sexual overtures
  - To counteract negative depictions and behavior toward them, nurses have reacted defensively and emotionally instead of carefully, convincingly, and competently

D. Healthcare Professionals and Patients Do Not View Patient Sexuality in the Same Way

Most patients enter the healthcare environment with some thoughts of foreboding, no matter how benign their illness. Their thoughts and concerns are primarily of their illness, the upcoming treatment, the potential for recovery or nonrecovery; the impact of the time and the possible procedures on many other personal factors, such as home, work, family, etc. Very little time initially is taken with thoughts and fantasies about their sexuality; however, this does not mean that the patient is asexual as some HCPs tend to believe.

1. **Patient Perceptions of Their Sexuality**
   - Many patients say they feel stripped and naked when they initially enter the healthcare environment, especially hospitals, not just from a shedding of clothing perspective but from an overall control perspective as well
   - Male patients at first feel as though they have been stripped of their maleness because they are no longer in charge, no longer seen as decision-makers, and often become passive, vulnerable, and helpless
   - The frequent niggling fear of castration that men sometimes envision outside of healthcare in one form or another (either figuratively or in actuality) becomes a very real threat, especially if surgery is indicated
   - When an HCP performs genital care on a male patient, it demeans him; he is mortified that another person, especially a female, should have to clean his penis, like a child. This again brings his sexuality into question
   - However, once the patients have overcome their initial fears, they often revert to the same patterns they usually

hold; however, probably not with the same frequency. They think about sex, fantasize about sex, and consider the physical attributes of those they see to whom they are sexually attracted
- Patients worry about the impact that the disease, hospitalization, and treatment may have on their future sex lives, and they ask themselves some of the following questions: "How disfiguring are the scars?" "When will I be able to have sex?" "How will my partner feel about sex now?" "Am I less sexually attractive?" "Will I be too tired to have sex?" "Will I be able to get an erection?" "Will I be able to be sexually aroused?" "Am I less feminine/masculine?" "Will I be the same?" "What about contraception?" "Will the pills interfere?" "Will sex hurt?" They would like to ask the HCP these questions, but they rarely do

2. **Healthcare Professionals' Perception and Acceptance of Patient Sexuality**
    - For the most part, HCPs treat all patients as being heterosexual (referred to as a heterocentrism script), and do not consider another sexual orientation
    - Same-sex sexual activities are especially difficult for HCPs to accept due to their inhibitions and internalized prejudices

Understanding Patients' Sexual Problems

- Patients who are homosexual or bisexual, are transgender, transsexual, or have a sex development variance, are sometimes confronted by HCPs who are rude, embarrassed, abrupt, verbally abusive, or who may ignore these patients completely. Patient responses to these situations vary according to the patients' feelings about their sexuality and the level of confidence in challenging the HCPs' unacceptable approach
- Patients may masturbate and also participate in other sexual activities with a partner while hospitalized; however, most HCPs do not recognize this and may not afford the patient the privacy he or she would like and deserves. The resulting behavior by some HCPs in response to patient sexual activities is giggling behind a hand, finger-pointing, and eye-rolling toward the heavens
- Some HCPs who work in a nursing home do not always acknowledge that residents are entitled to non-public sexual expression and privacy, as long as it is not self-harmful or harmful to others
- Rarely do HCPs say to patients "What questions do you have about your sexuality?" (Appendix B)

SECTION 2

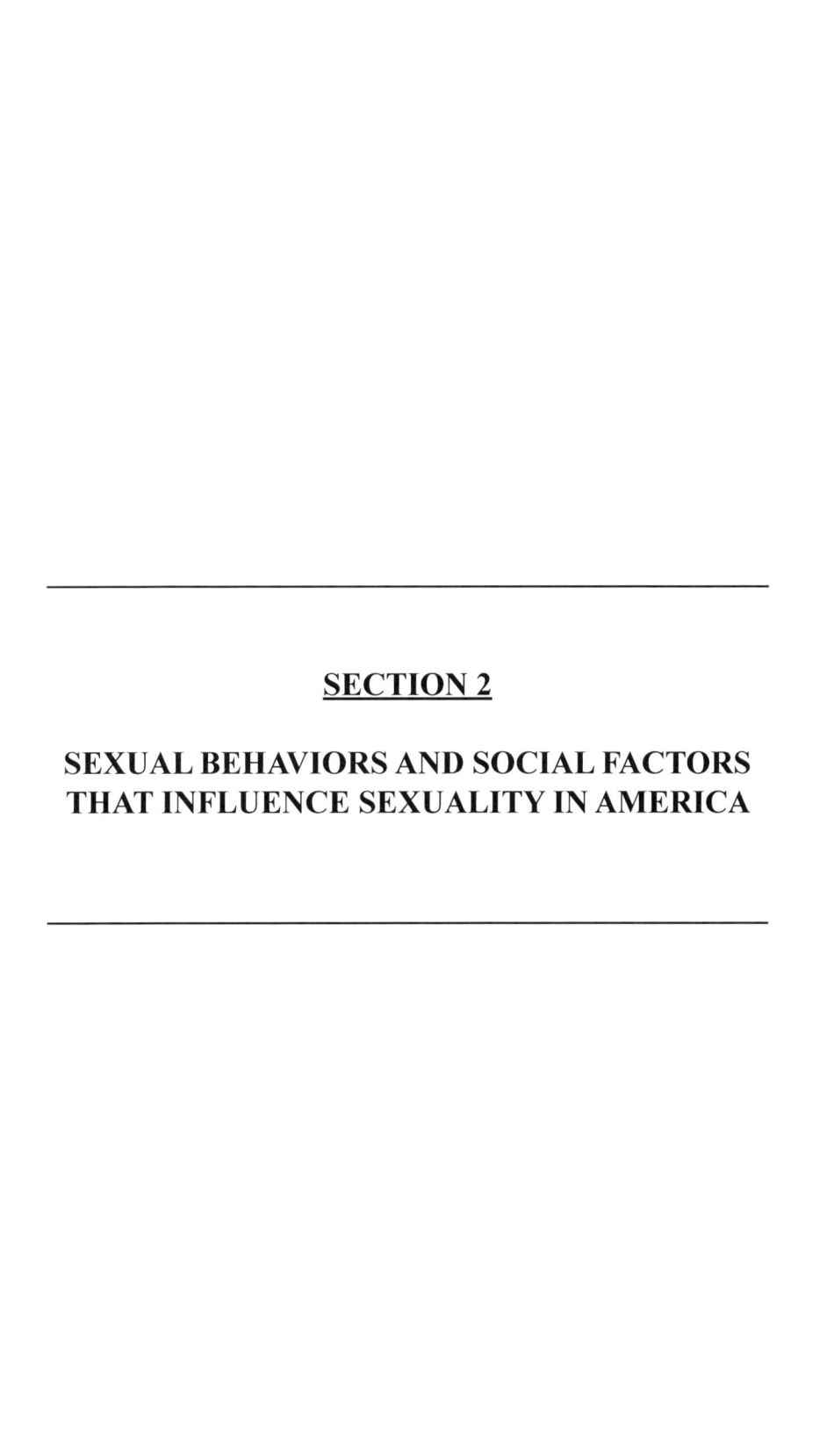

SEXUAL BEHAVIORS AND SOCIAL FACTORS THAT INFLUENCE SEXUALITY IN AMERICA

CHAPTER 2

SEXUAL BEHAVIORS AND TECHNIQUES ACCORDING TO A PERSON'S SEXUAL ORIENTATION

"I've oft been told by learned friars that wishing and the crime are one, and Heaven punishes desires as much as if the deed were done. If wishing damns us, you and I, are damned to all our heart's content. Come then, at least we may enjoy some pleasure for our punishment."

— Thomas Moore

Sexual orientation refers to an enduring pattern of emotional, romantic, and/or sexual attractions to men, women, or both; it also refers to a person's sense of identity based on those attractions, related behaviors, and membership in a community of others who share those attractions.[1] Sexual orientation is considered by most researchers to be fixed through life, and efforts to change one's sexual orientation usually fail. However, sexuality is also considered to be on a continuum, and sexual expression changes over time.

Understanding Patients' Sexual Problems

Although the use of labels is discouraged, most people use the following to identify a person's sexual orientation since it is easier than not to do so: *lesbians,* female homosexuals, are attracted to other women; *gay men,* male homosexuals, are attracted to other men; *bisexual* men and women are attracted to both men and women; and *asexuals* are not erotically or emotionally attracted to either sex.

Sexual Attraction and Sexual Orientation

Heterosexual males have a male physical body, with male genitalia (that they do not want to change), and a male gender identity. They are erotically and emotionally attracted to females (gynephilia).

Heterosexual females have a female physical body, female genitalia (which they do not wish to change), and female gender identity. They are erotically and emotionally attracted to males (androphilia).

Bisexual males and females are erotically and emotionally attracted to both males and females (biphilia). They may have a male or female gender identity according to their physical appearance and genitalia (which they do not want to change).

Homosexual males (androphilia) are emotionally, sexually, and physically attracted to other males, have a male physical body, and male genitalia (which they do not want to change), and a male gender identity. They are referred to as "gay men."

Homosexual females (gynephilia) are emotionally, sexually, and physically attracted to other women, have a female physical body, with female genitalia (which they do not want to change), and a female gender identity. They are referred to as "lesbians."

Asexual males and females self-identify as something other than homosexual or heterosexual; they are not sexually attracted to either gender; they are capable of sexual activities but have no desire or inclination. They are comfortable with their genitals.

Cross-dressers may be male or female, homosexual or heterosexual or bisexual. Many are male heterosexuals who express their femininity by wearing female clothing for comfort and erotically. They also use female mannerisms and gestures. A small group of females demonstrate their masculinity by wearing male clothing and use of male mannerisms and gestures. Both male and female cross-dressers are comfortable with their genitals.

Understanding Patients' Sexual Problems

Transgender males and females comprise a small group of people whose gender identity and physical body, sexual genitalia, and sexual orientation are not congruous. They are not usually comfortable with their genitals (may even hate them) and want them removed or changed.

Sexual Behaviors Enjoyed and Shared by People of Any Sexual Orientation. Sexual behaviors that those of any sexual orientation enjoy engaging in include kissing each other all over, deep French kissing, hugging, and overall body touching, initially without genital involvement, then later the genitals. Others are body massage, self and mutual masturbation (heavy petting), single and mutual oral sex (fellatio or cunnilingus), use of sex toys, and sexual experimentation, sexual sadism and masochism.

Heterosexual male sexual behaviors

- These behaviors are influenced by male heterosexual sexual and social scripts that propel the man toward being the hunter, chaser, and sex-initator, having casual sex, often taking the top and dominant position for intercourse, and valuing sexual pleasure. His sexual initiation, performance, prowess, and competence, penis size, and penile activities are of great importance
- Additional heterosexual male behaviors may include insertion of a finger into the female partner's vagina, insertion of penis into

Sexual Behaviors and Techniques

partner's vagina, and insertion of penis into female partner's anus

Heterosexual female sexual behaviors

- Female and heterosexual and social scripts influence heterosexual female behaviors. These heterosexual behaviors are being the hunted or the chased, valuing sex in a relationship, emotional jealousy, bottom (subservient) intercourse position, and defender or peacemaker
- Heterosexual female sexual behaviors (in addition to the previously mentioned general activities) also include reception of male partner's fingers into vagina, reception of male partner's penis into vagina, and reception of her male partner's penis into her anus

Homosexual male sexual behaviors

- Homosexual male sexual behaviors (in addition to the previously mentioned general sexual activities) also include receiving and giving male to male anal sex, *interfemoral* sex (penis thrusting in between partner's thighs), *rimming* (analingus, or tongue licking around partner's anus), and *fisting* (hand or arm inserted into male partner's anus; rare); the 69 position of anal and oral sex, and *frotting* (phallus to phallus, a male version of female frottage below)
- Anecdotally, there appears to be less emphasis on anal sex in actual

male homosexual sexual practice than portrayed in the popular media in which anal sex participation is usually exaggerated

> *"Males do not represent two discreet populations, heterosexual and homosexual. The world is not divided into sheep and goats: the living world is a continuum in each and every one of its aspects."*
>
> — Alfred Kinsey

Homosexual female sexual behaviors

- Homosexual female sexual behaviors (in addition to the previously mentioned general sexual activities) also include scissoring (vulva to vulva rubbing), which is an umbrella term for all types of frottage; fisting or the giving and receiving of female partner's fingers into vagina, nipple-sucking, clitoral stimulation, and sex toys, especially dildos
- In actual practice, less emphasis is given by lesbians to strapping a dildo and thrusting vaginally than is portrayed in the media. Instead, lesbians share a great deal of fantasy, support, intimacy, massage, and commitment in their relationships

> *"I was sixteen and my mother was about to throw me out of the house forever, for breaking a very big rule, even bigger than the forbidden books. The rule was not just*

No Sex, but Definitely No Sex with Your Own Sex."

— Jeanette Winterson

Lifestyles Based on Sexual Orientation

As previously mentioned, a person's sexual orientation, interest, and participation in a specific sexual behavior usually indicates the social circles or communities in which that person moves or lives, and the lifestyle adopted. The individual associates with others who share the same sexual interests and the groups they form tend to develop into actual communities. Some of the more frequent lifestyles and communities include bondage, discipline, sadism, and masochism (BDSM), bigamous, bisexual, and celibate, among others.

Non-Binary sexual identities and orientations (gender identities that do not fit within the societally created and accepted binary of male and female) also exist, including androphilia, gynephilia, pansexuality, polysexuality, third gender, and two spirit.

CHAPTER 3

THE SEXUAL PROCLIVITIES OF AMERICAN ADULTS, SOCIETAL MORES, AND THE MASS MEDIA'S IMPACT ON SEXUAL BEHAVIOR

"If Kinsey is right, I have only done what comes naturally, what the average American does secretly, drenching himself in guilt fixations and phobias because of his sense of sinning. I have never felt myself a sinner or committed what I call a sin."

— Mae West

When the words "sexual behavior" are mentioned, most people, especially heterosexuals, automatically envision sexual intercourse between two people. They do not always consider the many other sexual activities that are employed and enjoyed as part of many people's sexual expressions. Examples follow of some of these sexual techniques, behaviors, and associated activities that promote and enhance sexual pleasure.

Dreams (Sexual) and Emissions (Nocturnal or *Wet Dreams*)

Just as sexual fantasy is not actual sexual behavior, neither are sexual dreams. They do, however, act as a predictor of what sexual activities people might or might not want to participate in, and in so doing, may contribute to sexual arousal. Nocturnal emissions may or may not result from erotic dreams.

Points about Sexual Dreams and Nocturnal Emissions

- We dream because of the constant activity of our subconscious minds during sleep
- Freud in 1900 first wrote that "sexual dreams are attempts to fill desires that cannot be actualized during waking hours"[1]
- Some dreams are very erotic and may lead to arousal and orgasm during sleep and may wake the person
- Virtually all men and 70% of women have sexual dreams, although about only half of women have an orgasm during sleep."[2(p253)] The mind has a *dream censor* that, as its name implies, *cleans up* our dreams and replaces unacceptable images with those that are acceptable
- Wet dreams are so named because of the accompanying release of ejaculate
- Men between 21 and 25 years have the highest rate of nocturnal emission at 71%, and by the age of 50, this has

reduced to one-third, and by age 60, only 14% reported them; some men age 16 to 20 had 12 emissions per week, while others only a few a week.[3] Frequency varies, and it is usually more frequent in younger men
- Religions vary on their negative/positive attitudes toward nocturnal emissions.[4] For instance, some Asians believe that wet dreams are harmful, especially young Muslims. Most young Muslims, however, are taught to take a bath afterwards, and that a wet dream just makes one temporarily impure as it is an unconscious act, so not sinful
- In some parts of the world, nocturnal emission occurs more often than others; for instance, in Indonesia, 97% have experienced it before age 24.[4] Usually, the greater the frequency of masturbation, the lower the occurrence of nocturnal emissions

Fantasy (Sexual)

As with sexual dreams, sexual fantasy is not an actual sexual behavior; however, it is an extremely powerful tool that helps to induce sexual arousal, promote the desire, and at times reach orgasm.

"The best sex takes place in the mind first."

— Jenna Jameson

Understanding Patients' Sexual Problems

Points about Sexual Fantasy

- Contrary to common belief, sexual fantasies are healthy and occur most often in people with the fewest of sexual problems and least sexual dissatisfaction
- "54% of men think about sex every day or several times a day, 43% a few times a month, or a few times a week, and 4% less than once a month"[2 (p253)]
- "Nineteen percent of women fantasize every day or several times a day, 67% a few times a month, and 14% less than once a month"[2(p253)]
- The first sexual fantasy usually occurs between age 11 and 13, with men recalling earlier onset than women[2]
- Women who fantasize during masturbation are more likely to experience orgasm with intercourse, while men who fantasize often are more likely to achieve orgasm during intercourse[5]
- The majority of women fantasize, and fantasy is associated with greater sexual satisfaction of women as such fantasies may fulfill a beneficial role in their lives[5]
- Women fantasize about taking a passive role and being dominated during fantasy, men fantasize about being dominant, doing something sexual to their partners, or having multiple partners. Men's fantasies tend to be more sexually explicit than women's, and women's fantasies tend to be more emotional and romantic[6]

- Men fantasize an average of 7.2 times daily, and women 4.5 times daily[6]

"Man...heats up like a light bulb: red hot in the twinkling of an eye and cold again in a flash. The female, on the other hand... heats up like an iron. Slowly over a low heat, like tasty stew. But then, once she heats up there's no stopping her."

— Carlos Luis Zafoy

Flirting

Definition: Beach[7] described sexual attractiveness, proception, acception, and conception in female mammals as the process of sexual pairing. Proception is the courtship period during which non-human females secrete a pheromone from the vagina to which the male of the species is extremely sensitive; it remains questionable whether human females secrete similar pheromones. Flirting is a manifestation of proception, is most often and most successfully performed by women, and is used by women, through body language and verbal banter, to demonstrate interest in a potential mate.

Points about Flirting

- Flirting, as the proceptive phase, involves solicitation,

seduction, and attraction, and it is the phase before the acception phase when copulation occurs[7]
- The process includes verbal and non-verbal messages that convey being attracted to and feeling attractive
- Men appear to find flirting more difficult than women; many women are born flirts
- A woman frequently makes the first move in this process by looking pointedly at her target, walking toward the potential partner, swinging her hips, and thrusting her breasts toward the person of interest[8]
- Other behaviors include smiling, *chatting up* the target (with a tone of voice that indicates an interest), and a warm facial expression. A woman turns her body toward the target, tossing and touching her hair, licking her lips, and giving intermittent yet purposeful eye contact, among numerous other behaviors[8]
- The promise is usually that sex may be a possibility, but not a probability, and some men misconstrue some of the messages being sent; they confuse her friendliness with sexual availability[8]
- The process may advance or just *fizzle out*; however it ends, sexual feelings, thoughts, and desires have been stirred[8]

"Flirting is a woman's trade, one must keep in practice."

— Charlotte Brontë

Romantic and Limerent Love

Definition: Romantic love and limerent love are both positive motivators in the development of sexual attraction and sexual behaviors; however, they manifest themselves very differently. Romantic love (erotic love) has probably happened to most of us at one time or another, and it may or may not deepen to become a lasting, totally committed love. Occurring less frequently than romantic love is limerent love, a love that occurs in about 5% of the population.[9] This love can be manic, obsessive, dark, and all-consuming. When people are in the early stages of a romance, it is hard to distinguish *being in love* from *being in limerence*. However, as time goes on, it becomes easier to differentiate between the two; they start out somewhat the same, but play out very differently.

Points about romantic love

- Types of love described by Lewis[10] (from the Greek words) include *agape* (spiritual love), *storge* (affectionate love), *philos* (brotherly love), and *eros* (romantic love). Although Lewis described love from a Christian perspective, most religions describe love from a similar perspective
- Romantic love as described by Sternberg[11] also contains three elements: (a) passion with erotic attraction (feeling in love), (b) intimacy, closeness, connectedness, confiding, and (c)

commitment. Within these elements are seven types of love: liking-intimacy is high, but passion and commitment are low (usually called friendship); infatuation-passion is high but intimacy and commitment are low, often called "love at first sight"; empty love-commitment is high, but passion and intimacy are low, a "waning love or an arranged marriage," romantic love-intimacy and passion is high, but commitment is low, "Romeo and Juliet;" companionate love-intimacy and commitment are high, but passion is low, "passion has abated;" fatuous love-passion and commitment are high, but intimacy is low "whirlwind romance;" and consummate love—all three elements are present; "a love for which we all strive."[11(p276)]

- Western culture emphasizes romantic love as a prerequisite for marriage
- Romantic love is a universal or near universal human condition
- When people fall in love, they undergo three phases affected by their hormones: 1) The lust phase of new love is primed by the sex hormones, estrogen and progesterone; 2) the attraction (love-struck) phase is primed by norepinephrine, dopamine, and serotonin; and 3) the attachment phase is primed by vasopressin and oxytocin[11]

Points about limerent love

Tennov[12] first coined the term limerence as an involuntary interpersonal state that involves an acute longing for emotional reciprocation, obsessive-compulsive thoughts, feelings, and behaviors, and emotional dependence on another person. This intense interpersonal state is shown by such behaviors of affected individuals as:

- Idealization by the individuals of the love object (LO), with frequently occurring intrusive thoughts of that LO
- Excessive shyness, stuttering, nervousness, and confusion when in the presence of LO
- Fear of rejection and despair; even thoughts of suicide, if rejected
- Obsessive seeking of LO reciprocation, with excessive euphoria if it is reciprocated
- Maintenance of romantic intensity through any adversity
- A relationship that is unstable, intense, smothering, unrealistic, and unsatisfying
- Limerence is believed to be a mostly and obsessive-compulsive behavior disorder, with a 5% addiction component[9]

Masturbation

Masturbation Definition: The erotic stimulation of one's own or another's genitals to induce sexual arousal and frequently orgasm

Points about masturbation (according to Laumann[13(p81-84)])

- "...the better educated (some graduate school) are more likely to masturbate; 95 percent for men and 87 percent for women."
- The religiously conservative report lower rates than those with no religion. This difference suggests that more educated people are likely to have more secular views in general, have more liberal views of sexuality regardless of religion, and are more likely to think pleasure is a primary goal of sexual activity
- African-Americans report lower rates of masturbation than Caucasians
- The frequency of masturbation decreases in marriage, more for men than women, probably as a result of getting older
- There is no difference in masturbation of young women or older women living with a partner, or women who have never married
- The social scripting associated with masturbation is one of condemnation and guilt, about half of men and women who masturbate experience guilty feelings afterwards
- 63% of men and 42% of women currently masturbate
- People who have an active sex life are more likely than not to masturbate
- "Masturbation has the peculiar status of being highly

stigmatized and fairly commonplace."[13(p81)]
- Among married people, over half of husbands have masturbated in the past year, and over one-third of their wives have masturbated in the past year
- Masturbation is viewed by many as being something one does in the absence of available partners, not being sexually alluring to others, or being sexually incompetent

"Masturbation: the primary sexual activity of mankind. In the nineteenth century, it was a disease; in the twentieth, it's a cure."

— Thomas Szasz

Pornography

"I shall not today attempt further to define the kinds of material I understand to be embraced within that shorthand description ["hard-core pornography"], and perhaps I could never succeed in intelligibly doing so. But I know it when I see it...."

— Justice Potter Stewart

Definition: "Pornography is the representation in books, magazines, photographs, films, and other media of sexual behaviors that are erotic or lewd and are designed to arouse sexual interest."[14(p1)]

Points about pornography

- The First Amendment does not protect pornographic expression that corrupts people's behavior, and neither does it protect obscenity; consequently, pornography is limited to depictions of sexual behavior that must not be obscene[15]
- The Roth test states "whether to the average person, applying contemporary community standards, the dominant theme of the material appeals to a prurient (lewd or lustful) interest."[15] In 1967, the Supreme Court added that to establish obscenity, the material must also be "utterly without redeeming social value" and "patently offensive because it affronts contemporary community standards relating to the description of sexual matters"[15]
- In 1973, Justice Burger established three criteria that the material would need to meet to establish obscenity, including descriptions or representations of sex acts and masturbation, excretory functions, and lewd exhibition of the genitals[15]
- Berger also stated that only hardcore pornography could be designated as patently offensive
- The law also distinguishes between hard-core and soft-core pornography[15]
- Many radical feminists like MacKinnon[16] are vehemently opposed to pornography and compare the erotic images to an

instruction manual by which men are taught how to bind, batter, torture, and humiliate women
- Traditional conservatives and feminists also claim that viewing pornography causes women and children harm[16], and they believe that pornography is perverted, debases, harms, and objectifies women, and that all women in the sex trade are victimized
- Feminists also argue that pornography subordinates women, violates their right to equal civil status, and violates their civil right to freedom of speech. They also feel that pornography leads to an increase in rape, sexual assault, sexual harassment, prostitution, child molestation, and child sexual abuse
- Not all men become compulsive users of pornography; researchers estimate that only approximately 3-6% of users do so. Cooper[17] found that 8% used the Internet for more than 11 hours a week (heavy users), 45% used it for 1 to 10 hours a week (moderate users), and 46% used for less than one hour a week (low users)
- The Internet has made access to pornography easier; Cooper calls this the "Triple A-engine" effect, with accessibility, affordability, and anonymity[17]
- It appears that most viewing is done by men between their late teens and early adult years, with married men and churchmen abstaining more so than others. When women watch pornography, it is usually with their partners

- Some of the benefits of pornography are that it provides a legal outlet for illegal sexual activities, relieves anxiety and stress, decreases sex offenses (in particular child molestation), and improves the variety of sexual behaviors in long-term relationships
- When a man views pornography, his brain signals the release of chemical substances, endorphins, dopamine, and serotonin (pleasurable feelings), and sexual arousal, often accompanied by masturbation, follows. These pleasurable feelings result in the man wanting to repeat his viewing and masturbation behaviors[17]
- Excessive viewing of pornography has been reported to result in partner discord, divorce, family violence, broken homes, job loss, bankruptcy and loss of income, child molestation, sexual promiscuity, delinquency, perhaps incarceration, and ruined lives
- Pornography continues to be a heatedly debated topic in the U.S. One group argues that it is an acceptable sexual activity that benefits society, an act to which people cannot get addicted. Another group argues that it is not an acceptable sexual activity, people can and do become addicted, and it is a moral danger to society

Points about pornography that support that it is not an addiction

- Many psychologists doubt that addiction is the right term to use to describe what happens to people when they spend too much of their time watching pornography online.[18] Sexual compulsivity is suggested to be more appropriate
- Pornography as an addiction diagnosis was not included in the recent 2013 rewrite of the DSM-5 (fifth edition of the *Diagnostic and Statistical Manual of Mental Disorders*) by the American Psychological Association (APA) because of a lack of scientific evidence to support the claim that the viewing of pornography creates addicts
- There are no standard criteria for clinicians to diagnose viewing pornography as an addiction
- Ley in Brown[19] cautions clinicians that rather than helping patients who may struggle to control viewing images of a sexual nature, the 'porn addiction' concept instead seems to feed an industry with secondary gain from the acceptance of the idea
- Ley in Brown[19] also mentions that people who report pornography as an addiction are likely to be male, have a non-sexual (or asexual) orientation, have a high libido, tend toward sensation-seeking, and have religious values that conflict with their sexual behavior and desires

- Millions of men view porn and have no adverse consequences. Just as millions of people drink alcohol, but relatively few become alcoholics, so the same applies to watching pornography

Points about pornography that support that it is an addiction

- Voon[20], a Cambridge University (U.K.) neuropsychiatrist, has examined the brain activity patterns of men who view pornography to excess. So far, the brains of compulsive porn users resemble the brains of alcoholics watching ads for a drink. She also cautioned that there is insufficient evidence to advise about the impact of teenagers watching pornography on the Internet
- Therapists who treat pornography addicts say they behave just like any other addicts (gambling addicts, drug addicts)
- The signs and symptoms for men of viewing of pornography to excess are very similar to other addictions. These include total preoccupation with the behavior, an inability to manage that behavior (with numerous failed attempts to stop), marked personal distress about the behavior, family distress about the behavior
- The more pornography that addicts view, the more porn they need, and the more their sexual activities (and perhaps deviances) escalate, similar to other addictive behaviors seen in addicts
- In 2011, the American Society of Addiction Medicine[21]

(ASAM) defined addiction for the first time and included that addiction includes pathological pursuit of all kinds of external rewards and not just substance dependence. It does not explicitly include porn addiction
- ASAM[21] unequivocally states "behavior addictions involve similar alterations and neural pathways as do drug addictions. We believe Internet porn should not be under the sex addiction umbrella."
- Kruger[22] (a psychiatrist member of the DSM-5 group to consider sex as an addiction) has said he has little doubt that porn addiction is real and will eventually garner enough attention to be recognized as a mental illness by the DSM. However, Krueger also warns that the kind of definitive research that explains what happens to the brain by watching porn has yet to be done

Points for Discussion:

What makes you believe or not believe that pornography is an addiction?

Why do you agree or disagree that pornography is a danger to society?

"Consuming pornography does not promote sex if one defines sex as a shared act between two partners. It promotes masturbation. It promotes the solitary auto-arousal that precludes intimacy and love. Pornography is about getting yourself off at someone else's expense."

— Chris Hedges

Prostitution

Definition: A New Mexico statute indicates that "Prostitution consists of knowingly engaging in or offering to engage in a sexual act for hire. Sexual act means sexual intercourse, cunnilingus, fellatio, masturbation of another, anal intercourse or the causing of penetration to any extent and with any object of the genital or anal opening of another, whether or not there is any emission. Whoever commits prostitution is guilty of a petty misdemeanor, unless such crime is a second or subsequent conviction, in which case such a person is guilty of a misdemeanor."[23] A prostitute is a woman who engages in sexual intercourse for money, a man who engages in such activity, especially in homosexual practices, and a person who offers his talent or work for unworthy purposes[24]

Points about prostitution

- Prostitution is said to be the oldest profession in the world (untrue), an expression used as a way to convey that prostitution has been around for thousands of years and, therefore, is a viable commodity
- Prostitution is present within all social strata, and it exists as a response to societal demand
- The life of a prostitute had not changed a great deal since Victorian times until recently with the advent of the Internet
- The well-kept, high-priced call girl has replaced the Victorian mistress while some average prostitutes (hookers or working girls) still walk the streets, but a middle man (pimp) may still be in the picture, to protect his girls
- Prostitutes have been moved off the streets in many cities in response to public outcries about their high visibility in public. The luckier ones have moved into shabby hotel rooms or apartments, while the unlucky ones remain on the streets to perform cheap *tricks* in dark alleys like their predecessors
- The Internet has improved the lives of prostitutes in a number of ways so more women have chosen prostitution as a career path. The Internet has increased their independence through increased and timely access to customers, choice of their own hours according to appointments, shorter work weeks, and less need to work for a pimp.[25] "Craigslist didn't just lower

the barriers to entry for sex workers and clients—it all but eliminated them."

For many years, an ongoing debate has existed between those who believe prostitution is a victimless crime, so it should be decriminalized and legalized, and those who feel prostitution is a crime and should remain classified as a criminal act.

Support of Decriminalization, Regulation, and Legalization of Prostitution

- Prostitution is an act between consenting adults and provides a service
- Prostitution is a victimless crime
- Prostitution is an exchange of money for the service, just like any other financial transaction
- Women and men choose to enter the *profession* of prostitution as the best job alternative available to them; primarily an economic decision
- Legalization and regulation will ensure testing prostitutes for STIs and HIV
- Decriminalization will provide protection from the police instead of their current arresting of prostitutes
- Sex trafficking, rape, and sexual coercion will be reduced if prostitution is decriminalized

- Sex should be freely distributed just like any other service

Non-Support of Decriminalization, Regulation, and Legalization of Prostitution

- Prostitutes, adolescent men, women, and children are all victims of coercion, fear, and violence
- The services that prostitutes have to provide include being raped, sodomized, whipped, bound, and gagged
- Non-supporters of decriminalization claim prostitution is immoral. It is questionable whether this claim is for religious reasons or a human rights issue
- Just because it is the world's oldest profession does not make prostitution moral
- Women choose prostitution over poverty; they are between *a rock and a hard place*
- Testing for HIV does not provide protection because people test as negative for three months after exposure
- Men who rape wives will continue to do so; rape is about control, not sex
- Most women consent to sex under pressure from the *john* or pimp

Points for Discussion:

How is prostitution an immoral act?

Why do you believe or not believe that prostitution should be decriminalized and legalized?

Why do you believe or not believe prostitution performs a needed service within society?

If prostitution were decriminalized, how would this impact rapes and sexual assaults?

Sexual Scripting

Definition: Sexual Scripting[26] (also referred to as Sexual Socialization) is a social and cultural process that involves observation and the imitation of witnessed sexual behaviors (behavior modeling) of people, marketing outputs, the written word, and the entertainment media. According to the theory first proposed in 1973 by Gagnon and Simon (and elaborated upon in 1987), at birth we are blank slates, with little or no understanding about how to behave sexually; we learn about and add sexuality data to our slate as we go along.

Points about Sexual Scripting

- The learning process, the blueprint of our sexuality, is passive and unintentional
- These blueprints are individual-specific; however, some of these individual blueprints have become the standard for sexual behavior within a given society, and many of them are often detrimental to healthy sexual behavior
- Sexual scripts provide direction about how to act, think, progress, respond, and feel in sexual situations, as well as influence psychosexual development of both sexes
- The person's upbringing, as well as social factors such as gender roles, class, ethnicity, education, and religion play a

Understanding Patients' Sexual Problems

   great part in sexual scripting
- Fantasy (as a type of script) is a frequently used method for arousal; it works, and most American adults do it
- Scripting of men's fantasies are mostly explicitly sexual and aggressive; women's feature romance
- The heterosexual script is that men are expected to initiate and guide sexual activity and be decisive and knowledgeable about sexual activity. Women are expected to be passive, compliant with the initiation of sexual activity, and responsive and pleased with a sexual encounter as it progresses[27]
- Male sexual scripts also include control, casual relationships, being the aggressor in sex, being assertive, being promiscuous, initiating, competitive, and performance-oriented; a woman's orgasm indicates male success
- Female sexual scripts include being submissive, passive, sexually responsive, resistive, seductive, the non-initiator of sex, loving, and committed to relationships
- Many heterosexual fantasies envision intercourse with a same-sex partner, but this does not indicate that the person has a homosexual orientation

SECTION 3

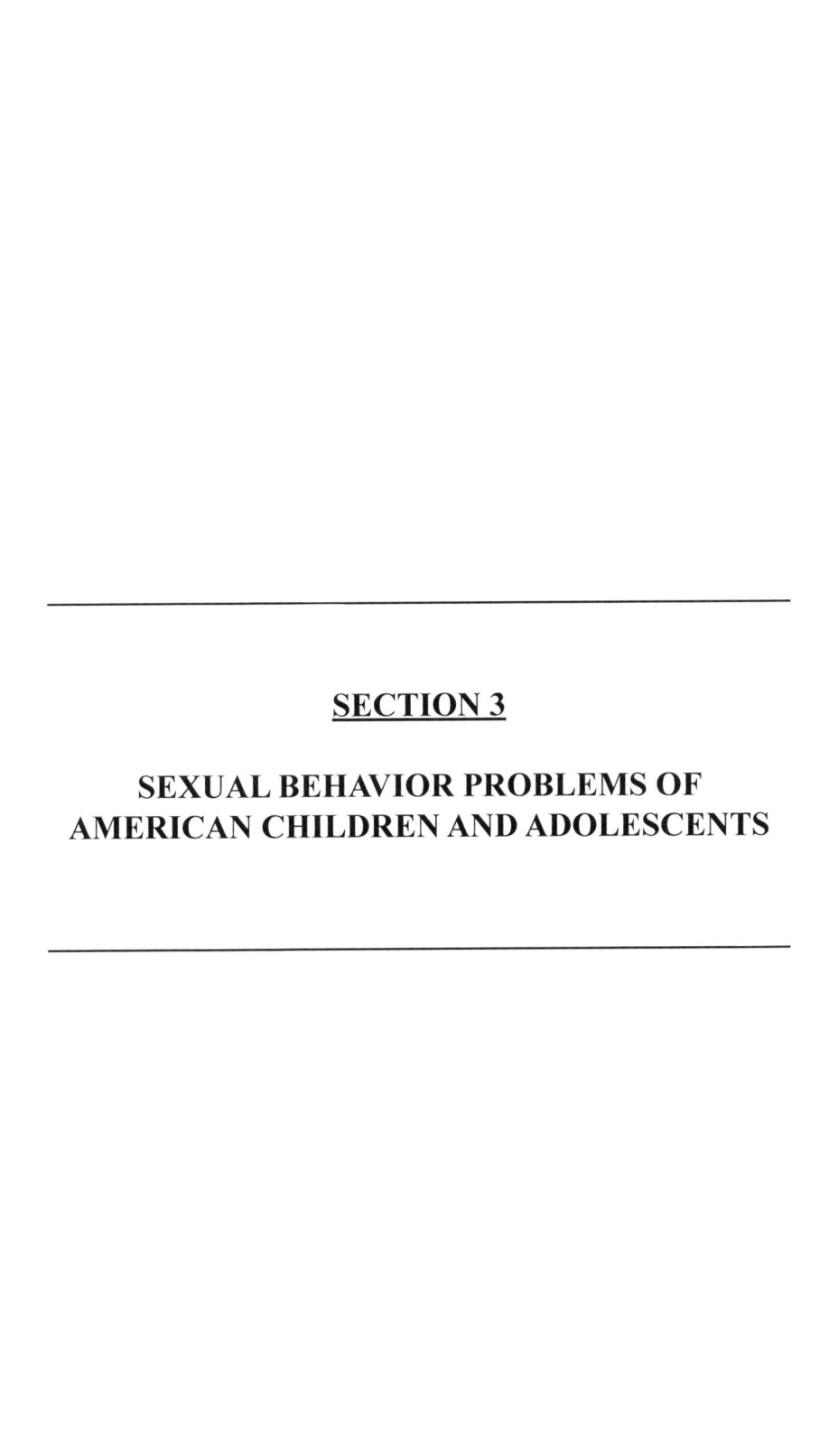

SEXUAL BEHAVIOR PROBLEMS OF AMERICAN CHILDREN AND ADOLESCENTS

CHAPTER 4

DIFFERENTIATING BETWEEN EXPECTED CHILDHOOD CURIOSITY AND UNEXPECTED SEXUAL BEHAVIOR PROBLEMS OF CHILDREN

"Victims of harmful sexual behaviour may not know that what has been done to them is wrong, especially if it is seen as normal among their peers."

— Ringrose, J. NSPCCC (U.K.)

For a young child to emerge from childhood with a healthy perception of sexuality might seem to be almost impossible. However, most children do so successfully, and they go on to adulthood to have healthy, productive, and meaningful sexual lives. Even children who are the recipients of some sex-negative attitudes in Western culture usually overcome this negative outlook and grow into sexually satisfied adults. Unfortunately, this positive outcome is not achieved by all children; some have to overcome many obstacles toward healthy adult sexuality during their formative years.

Some obstacles to healthy childhood sexuality include: 1) The sexualization of young girls; 2) gender dysphoria in children; 3) sexual developmental differences or variances in children, which include: 3a) Turner syndrome, 3b) Klinefelter syndrome, 3c) XXY syndrome, and 3d) XYY syndrome; 4) androgen insufficiency to include: 4a) complete androgen insufficiency, 4b) partial androgen insufficiency, and 4c) mild androgen insufficiency; 5) hypospadias; 6) cryptorchidism; 7) congenital adrenal hyperplasia; 8) child sexual abuse; 9) sexual behavior problems in children; 10) female genital cutting; and 11) sexually transmitted infections in children. We'll look at each of these in more detail.

1. The Sexualization of Young American Girls

The sexualization process of young and adolescent girls usually begins when they are quite young; it begins slowly and is barely noticeable, and it continues as they approach womanhood. Openly suggestive advertisements in sexual videos, movies, television, and magazines surround young girls who are forced to participate in "tots" beauty pageants by overly-eager mothers, are moulded by multitudes of societal pressures, and come into contact with people who value them for their sexiness rather than their personalities until the young women finally acquiesce. Young and adolescent girls come to believe that being attractive equates to being sexy, and being sexy becomes a measure of their self-worth. They begin to act sexually and become marked sexual targets for some men who perceive them to be older, sexually knowledgeable, and sexually available. In the U.S., girls are surrounded and influenced by the prevailing sexually charged environment that forces sexually-explicit information on young, easily influenced children.

A. **Definition.** Sexualization is the process by which a young person (primarily a girl) is encouraged to become sexual, is valued by society for being sexy, becomes sexually objectified by others, either as an individual or as a group, and measures her own worth accordingly.

B. **Signs and Symptoms**

- Girls and young women routinely wear sexually provocative, age-inappropriate clothing, with an excessive amount of makeup and jewelry. They use hair extensions and false eyelashes in their attempts to increase their overall sexiness, sexualize their appearance, and promote sex appeal, and thereby, gain acceptance
- A young girl's behavior becomes flirtatious and sexually suggestive, with sexual posturing, sexual gestures, and sexual mannerisms
- Girls and young women believe that physical attractiveness and sex appeal are the same

- The girl looks much older than her actual age, which suggests, especially to men, a sexual awareness and sexual experience far beyond her years, as well as indicates availability for sexual exploitation

C. Origins

- Sexualization occurs when a young girl's self-value comes from her sexual appeal to the exclusion of all other characteristics, when physical attractiveness equates to being sexy, when she is sexually objectified, and when sexuality is inappropriately imposed upon her. All four conditions need not be present at the same time[1(p1)]
- The majority of mainstream media in the U.S. sexualizes children and young women through overt and covert marketing advertisements on television, radio, print, billboards, and sports-related events. Girls and women are sex objects in movies, television programs, music videos, cartoons, video games, music lyrics, etc.
- Cartoons for young girls that show the heroine with low cleavage, age-inappropriate clothing, adult mannerisms, provocative speech, and as the receiver of sexist remarks by male figures
- Sexually explicit *pop-music* videos in which girls do nothing to add artistic value, but just stand around to

provide *eye candy* for male viewers. Meanwhile, the songs are full of denigrating lyrics written and sung by males
- Sexualization may be imposed on a young girl by her mother (or another female with influence over the young girl), or by other members of the girl's family. The girl is pressured to appear in child beauty pageants where the girl is dressed to imitate looking like a woman, with all the associated *trappings* and encouraged to walk, talk, and act older than her young years[1(p15)]

D. Background

- Most young American girls are adversely impacted by the presence of the dominant culture that exists around them, regardless of their ethnicity. However, often additional sexual stereotypes are imposed upon girls from different ethnic, socio-economic, religious, and family backgrounds, as well as among girls of different sexual orientations[1(p15)]
- The sexuality of a young girl is valued more highly in American society than her academic, sports, artistic, and community achievements
- The perception by a girl that her physical appearance (thinness, *bustiness*, and sexiness) are more valued by others than her many other attributes

- According to Nichter,[2] "African-American girls received more positive feedback about their appearance from their parents that resulted in greater body satisfaction and self-esteem and less concern about their weight."

E. Therapeutic Interventions

- Perform a Standard Sexual Assessment (Appendix C), a medical assessment, and obtain sexual and medical histories
- Participate in community-wide efforts to reduce the sexualization of girls and young women
- "Encourage girls to focus on body competence instead of body appearance; participation in physical activity may be one of girls' best means of resisting objectification and sexualization"[1 (p35)]
- Evaluate the girl for signs of sexual knowledge, sexual experience, and sexual provocativeness beyond her stated age. Observe for evidence of sexual abuse (see child sexual abuse section), her relationship with her parents, siblings, peers, and adult males
- Refer the girl for psychiatric support if depression or the potential for self-injury occur

Unexpected Sexual Behaviors

F. Supportive Interventions

- Review the Guidelines for Supportive Interventions for Children (Appendix G)
- Provide comprehensive sexual education that includes accurate and current information about contraception, reproduction, self-image, and self-esteem, as well as sexual abstinence and comprehensive sexual education (abstinence alone without comprehensive education is not effective)
- Include communication skills that enhance the girl's ability to say, "No" to a boy's sexual requests or demands
- Describe to the girl the adverse impact that the media has on her sexuality, and facilitate media education to increase her awareness
- Encourage increased participation in physical activity to promote positive mood and feelings of confidence[1(p21)]
- Educate and enlist the support and assistance of the girl's parents to promote other attributes in their child and reduce the chance of further sexualization
- If the mother insists on her daughter's beauty pageant participation in spite of her child's potential sexualization, provide appropriate education. If not effective, refer to a pediatric nurse practitioner or physician

G. Potential Outcomes

- "There is evidence that sexualization contributes to impaired cognitive performance in college-aged women…. Viewing material that is sexually objectifying can contribute to body dissatisfaction, low self-esteem, depressive effect, and even physical health problems in high-school aged girls and in young women" [1(p2)]
- Girls who are sexualized are easy prey for people (predominantly) men who procure them for their enjoyment and force girls into drug use, prostitution, and sex-trafficking
- Self-objectification in young girls leads to poor sexual health, such as eating issues, depression, and isolation

2. Gender Identity Dysphoria in Children

The treatment of gender identity dysphoria in children (GIDIC) is more controversial and difficult than in adults because children have a limited verbal capacity with which to express their needs, desires, or what they understand. They do not possess the cognitive skills needed to make decisions about the treatment of their gender identity. According to Zucker[3(p4)] "There is a dearth of randomized controlled treatment outcome studies of children who present with GIDIC." Consequently, informed decisions are difficult to make.

A. **Definition.** Gender dysphoria (GD) in children is a term used to describe children who experience a marked difference between their expressed/experienced gender and the gender assigned by others at birth; this difference must be present for at least six months. This condition causes clinically significant distress or impairment in social, occupational, or other important areas of functioning[4]

B. Signs and Symptoms

- Feelings of incongruence between a child's felt gender identity and his or her primary and secondary sex characteristics, with a desire by the child to eliminate his or her primary and secondary sex characteristics; in children, there must be a desire to be of the other gender, and this desire actually verbalized[4]
- The child believes he or she has the feelings and reactions typical of the other sex, the individual does not have a sexual development variance, and the condition causes significant distress in the child
- The child expresses a desire to be the opposite sex

(including passing as the opposite sex and calling self by an opposite sex name)
- The child expresses disgust with his or her genitals; a boy may pretend he does not have a penis
- Girls may fear growing breasts and menstruation, may bind their breasts, and may refuse to sit when urinating
- The child believes he or she will grow up to be the opposite sex
- Is rejected, ostracized, and bullied by their peers
- Dresses and behaves in a manner typical of the opposite sex
- Experiences such feelings as isolation, depression, and anxiety,[5] as well as manifestations of low self-esteem, fear, anger, self-blame and shame, disruptive behavior, sadness, and depression

C. Origins

- The exact origin of gender identity dysphoria has not been identified, but many theories have been proposed. These include a) internal influences within the fetus very early in utero (nature, biology), b) influences that occur in the child after birth (nurture, environment), and/or c) internal biological influences that interact with external environmental influences

Unexpected Sexual Behaviors

- "The exact cause of gender dysphoria is not known, but several theories exist. These theories suggest that the disorder may be caused by genetic (inherited) abnormalities, hormone imbalances during fetal and childhood development, defects in normal human bonding and child rearing, or a combination of these factors."[5 (p1)]

D. Background

- Gender dysphoria is experienced by children of all races, cultures, religions, or socio-economic status, has existed for many hundreds of years, and was received with more tolerance in previous centuries than in current times
- Gender variance is not rare, but transsexualism is, and most children do not become transsexual adults; they go on to identify as heterosexual, homosexual (most frequent), bisexual, asexual, non-gendered, or of a blended gender
- The child is aware of differences between self and other children at age three to five; the result is an unhappy, confused, lonely, and depressed child as he or she attempts to conform to societal pressures and understand his or her own inner feelings

- The initial response from many parents may be denial, embarrassment, shame, fear, and grief; followed by either acceptance, support, or continued denial, especially by the father of a son who believes he is a girl
- Often ostracized, bullied, and ridiculed at school, the child finds puberty an unbearable time

E. Therapeutic Interventions

- Perform a Standard Sexual Assessment (Appendix C) and a medical assessment, and obtain a sexual and medical history
- Involve all needed expert HCPs, such as a psychiatrist, a psychologist, a psychiatric nurse practitioner, and geneticist
- Three standard treatment pathways for the treatment of GD currently exist, one of which is selected by the physician based upon his or her experiences, knowledge, past successes, and beliefs:
  a) Encourage the child to become more congruent with the gender assigned at birth, and encourage the use of gender-assigned, gender identity conforming behaviors, OR
  b) Discourage the child from becoming more congruent with gender identity assigned at birth

and discourage the use of gender-assigned gender identity conforming behaviors, OR

c) Maintain the child with a neutral gender identity until he or she attains an age when more able to make his or her own decision with regards to gender identity

- Other infrequently used interventions that the physician, parents, and child may decide upon is to allow the child to go through the natural pubertal process uninterrupted (which may cause the child distress due to the sometimes extreme body changes that occur), OR suspend the child's puberty through hormonal intervention and stop those hormones at about age 16
- Over the past ten years or so, and extremely rarely, physicians in the Netherlands and the U.S. have performed sex reassignment on children younger than age 18; this remains controversial
- Prescribe all necessary interventions from childhood through adulthood, to include medications that support treatment pathway interventions
- Obtain expert consultations on any psychological issues, school issues, appearance issues, pubertal issues, associated medical issues, relationship issues

F. Supportive Interventions

- Review the Supportive Interventions Guide for Children (Appendix G)
- Either be in agreement with the medical practitioners treatment pathway selected for a child or decline to become involved in the process due to ethical considerations
- Visually assess the child's behavior, socialization, affect, interaction with parents, caregivers, and other children; preferred toys, play activities, etc.
- Evaluate the child's understanding of the decided upon treatment and his or her perceptions of what the particular pathway includes and what it means to the child
- Implement the selected treatment method, either a), b), or c) as determined by a physician and the team
- According to Spiegel,[6(p2)] "The majority of therapists currently employ these techniques" (to discourage the child from becoming more congruent with the gender assigned at birth and discourage the use of gender-assigned, gender identity conforming behaviors), "even though this approach causes the child anguish due to the withdrawal of praise and addition of penalties for all non-gender assigned behaviors"

Unexpected Sexual Behaviors

- Observe for any manifestations of low self-esteem, fear, anger, self-blame and shame, anxiety, disruptive behavior, anxiety, sadness, and depression

G. Potential Outcomes

- In a study by Wallien and Cohen-Kettenis[7] of 77 children (59 boys and 18 girls) in 2008, 12 boys and 8 girls still identified after puberty as having GID (*persistence* group); nearly all of the males and females in this group of 20 children identified as being homosexual or bisexual. Of those in the *desistence* group, all the girls and half the boys identified as being heterosexual, while the other half of the boys identified as being homosexual or bisexual
- Of the children who are untreated, a small minority will identify as being transsexual. Most become comfortable with their natal gender over time and are classified in the desistence group
- A small group of children become adults who will choose to do one of a few things: nothing at all, cross-dress into their desired sex, take hormonal therapy to change to their desired sex without transition surgery, or take hormonal therapy and transition surgery to change to their desired sex

"John [the father] kept saying, 'You have a penis. That means you are a boy.' One day, Shannon noticed that her son had been in the bathroom an awfully long time and pushed the door open. 'He had a pair of my best, sharpest sewing scissors poised, ready to cut. Penis in the scissors. I said, 'What are you doing?' He said, 'This doesn't belong here. So I'm going to cut it off.' I said, 'You can't do that.' He said, 'Why not? 'I said, 'Because if you ever want to have girl parts, they need that to make them.' I pulled that one right out of my ass. He handed me the scissors and said, 'Okay.'"

— Andrew Soloman

3. Sexual Developmental Incongruence in Children

"We can't ignore right-wing demagogues who insist that the word of the doctor who proclaims a child's sex at birth somehow holds more sway over the reality of the body than the word of the person who inhabits it."

— Kate Bornstein

Biological sex is determined by an assortment of factors—the number of and types of sex chromosomes, the type of gonads (ovaries or testicles), the sex hormones, the internal reproductive anatomy, and the external genitalia. Sexual variations exist in a fetus when the usual pathway or activity involved in sexual development is not taken and, as a result, the fetus may have a chromosomal, gonadal and/or bodily appearance that is atypical. According to Diamond, quite possibly the world's leading expert in sex development incongruence, "About 1 child in every 2,000 is born with enough ambiguity that it's externally noticeable. One in every 100 has hidden ambiguity—XXY or other sets of chromosomes or combinations of ovaries and testes."[8(p1)]

The biological sex of a fetus is determined by the presence or absence of the Y-linked gene, SRY, in that a fetus with at least one Y chromosome develops as male. Signs and symptoms of X and Y chromosome variations differ according to the number of X and Y chromosomes present in the child's cells. Management of chromosomal variations in a child is determined by the type of pattern present within the child's cells, the clinical picture with which the child presents, and the child's identified needs. The most frequently occurring chromosomal syndromes are Turner syndrome and Klinefelter syndrome, followed by XYY syndrome, and XXX syndrome.

3a. Turner Syndrome (45,X /44XO)

A. Definition. A chromosomal variance that only affects females in which there is a missing or incomplete sex chromosome. This variance may lead to some aspects of non-standard or variant anatomical, neurological, and sexual development in an infant girl.[9]

B. Signs and Symptoms

- Inwardly the child feels like a girl and outwardly looks like a girl. Short stature, with a round face, puffy hands and feet, enlarged breasts with a broad chest. Develops sexually, has a uterus but may have no vagina, lacks typical ovaries but has ovarian *streaks* instead
- External genitalia appear mostly normal
- No sex hormones, does not experience puberty, is usually infertile, and does not menstruate
- May have cardiac, renal, auditory, thyroid, and skeletal anomalies (scoliosis, osteoporosis)[9]
- Socially integrated, with average intelligence, but has the potential for problems with math, memory, and attention
- Over-compliant, timid, motherly, with delayed emotional maturity
- May have loose neck skin and neck webbing; low set ears, and many moles[9]

C. Origins

- The child's Y sex chromosome is usually missing or the child has only a partial Y chromosome
- May have a single X chromosome, with or without mosaicism (where cells have an abnormal number of chromosomes while others may have an extra chromosome)
- Actual cause of the missing Y chromosome is unknown

D. Background

- Usually diagnosed at or after puberty when expected menstruation fails to occur
- Increased morbidity/mortality at slightly earlier age
- Affects 1 in 2,000 female births, with a high fetal death rate during the mother's first trimester; approximately 70,000 women and girls in the U.S. today have this condition[9]
- Reared as girls

E. Therapeutic Interventions

- Perform a Standard Sexual Assessment (Appendix

C) and medical assessment and obtain a sexual history from parents, especially history of contributing factors
- Refer to a pediatric geneticist, endocrinologist, speech therapist, physical therapist, cardiologist, teachers, nurse practitioner, and a psychologist
- Diagnostics include amniocentesis while in utero, an MRI, ultrasound of pelvis, and karyotype (chromosome analysis)
- Institute hormone and androgen regime to stimulate growth, estrogens to develop breast tissue, and promote other secondary sex characteristics
- Prepare the child for puberty and the young woman for pregnancy (if she desires)
- Monitor and treat any associated medical conditions
- Develop long range plans, and plan to see the child at least quarterly until stable

F. Supportive Interventions

- Review Supportive Interventions Guide for Children (Appendix G)
- Monitor attendance of the child at the clinic to ensure continuity of care
- Observe for issues with memory, school per-

formance, and socialization
- Administer growth hormones to the child to increase height, estrogens for secondary sex characteristics, and estrogens and progesterone to help child move toward puberty and menses. Monitor growth parameters
- Prepare for and assist physician and child during procedures
- Provide counseling to the child if she has inadequate relationships and low self-esteem
- Provide support, education, and reassurance to the child and the parents
- Monitor routinely for cardiac and kidney complications, elevated blood pressure, diabetes, obesity, scoliosis, hip displacement, hearing issues, among other potential symptoms
- No elective genital surgery is indicated

G. Potential Outcomes

- No cure; however, most girls with Turner syndrome who have hormone treatment lead normal, happy, and healthy lives, with pregnancy sometimes possible through medical intervention

3b. Klinefelter Syndrome (47,XXY)

A. Definition. A chromosomal variance that only affects males in which there is at least one extra female sex chromosome present at the cellular level. This chromosomal variance leads to some aspects of non-standard anatomical, neurological, endocrine, and sexual development in the infant boy.

B. Signs and Symptoms

- Normal at birth, with average birth weight and size, and normal genitalia, yet becomes tall for his age later
- Boys are anatomically male, with a small penis due to lack of testosterone
- Genitals may not virilize at puberty, but internal sex organs are standard. Body changes occur fairly radically at puberty, following which anger and rage may flare with the least provocation and frustration
- May also have cryptorchidism (undescended testes) and hypospadias (a urethral opening on the underside of the shaft of the penis)[10]
- Sparse hair distribution, and may have female body shape, large breasts, increased incidence of breast cancer, and infertility

- May have speech issues and learning difficulties; however, some may have above average academic abilities

C. Origins

- Male has an extra X sex chromosome, so XXY configuration. If more X chromosomes present, 48,XXXY or 49,XXXXY, the boy's signs and symptoms are often more severe
- 60% of embryos with Klinefelter syndrome do not survive the fetal period[10]
- Not inherited, and risk of occurring again in another pregnancy not greater than in the general population

D. Background

- Condition often not diagnosed until after puberty
- One of the most frequent chromosomal abnormalities, and affects 1 in 500-800 births, with 3,000 affected boys born each year; impacts all racial and ethnic groups equally[10]
- Frequently underdiagnosed as the mild form often missed. Not inherited, random

- Reared as boys

E. Therapeutic Interventions

- Perform Standard Sexual Assessment (Appendix C) and medical assessment, and obtain sexual and medical history from parents, especially history of contributing factors
- Early assessment and involvement of a pediatric endocrinologist, a developmental psychologist, and a speech therapist, and perhaps an anger management therapist
- Begin long-term testosterone therapy at puberty to alleviate low sex drive and reduce feminine aspects of behavior and appearance
- Breast reduction/removal surgery
- Early elective genital surgery not indicated

F. Supportive Interventions

- Review the Supportive Interventions Guide for Children (Appendix G)
- Educate child (when appropriate) and parents about genetic differences
- Manage child's anger outbursts and tendency to

violence; observe/teach safety precautions to child and family
- Educate regarding all medications, especially testosterone, and treatment protocols; check with parents for compliance
- Monitor speech and learning disorders, and refer to speech therapist
- Determine child's awareness of changes that occur during puberty, and prepare him accordingly
- Observe for psychological issues and obtain expert interventions

G. Potential Outcomes

- There is no known cure for chromosome variances; however, some increased X chromosome symptoms may be alleviated with testosterone
- Majority of males with a mild case will lead standard, productive lives but may have a shortened lifespan
- Most will be sterile
- A small percentage of boys may have associated diseases and emotional/psychological issues

Note: Boys with an XYY chromosomal pattern

(below) have similar but fewer signs and symptoms to boys with Klinefelter syndrome, but are often classified together

3c. XYY Syndrome

A. Definition. A genetic condition in which there is an extra Y chromosome in all or many of the boy's cells. (This extra Y chromosome results in a condition that is somewhat similar to Klinefelter syndrome described previously.) The effects of an extra Y chromosome depend on the proportion of XY cells to XYY cells.

B. Signs and Symptoms

- No visible differences at birth. Overall, they are calm babies and caring, gentle children
- Weak muscle tone as a baby, and slow with crawling and walking. Some slowness in development, especially speech and language
- Some learning difficulties,[11] but due to size, expected to perform at better level; with some behavioral and emotional issues
- Delayed or absent puberty with undescended testicles and low testosterone levels

C. Origins

- Extra Y chromosome in some cells, with some XY cells present
- Not inherited, random

D. Background

- Occurs in 1 in 1,000 boys,[11] and most never know they have this condition as it is not routine to have every baby's chromosomes checked
- The boys have normal intelligence, although they are often expected to be advanced for their age because they are taller for their age
- Reared as boys; normal puberty

E. Therapeutic Interventions

- Perform Standard Sexual Assessment (Appendix C) and medical assessment, and obtain a sexual and medical history from parents, especially history of contributing factors
- Assess early and involve pediatric geneticist, speech therapist, physical therapist, a pediatric surgeon, and teachers

- Initiate testosterone and surgery to release testes. Monitor through childhood
- No elective genital surgery required

F. Supportive Interventions

- Review the Supportive Interventions Guide for Children (Appendix G)
- Provide a range of motion exercises, and assist the child with crawling and walking; reinforce physical and occupational therapy
- Educate parents and child regarding XYY syndrome
- Administer and explain all aspects of testosterone therapy
- Provide routine post-operative testes release care

G. Potential Outcomes

- The majority of boys with XYY lead happy, healthy, and productive lives[12]
- Most speech and ambulation issues usually resolve relatively quickly

3d. Triple X Syndrome (47,XXX)

A. Definition. A sex chromosomal abnormality in which a baby girl is born with a genetic karyotype of 47,XXX not expected prior to her birth. Most have no issues of which they are aware.

B. Signs and Symptoms

- Fetus develops as a female as there is no Y chromosome present[13]
- May have slow growth, low I.Q., or physical and developmental issues while at school, but the young woman does fairly well after school completion
- Psychiatric disorders occur fairly frequently
- Born with a low birth weight and a small head circumference
- May have genital anomalies, seizures, kidney issues
- MRIs show decreased brain volumes, and EEG abnormalities are relatively common
- Some verbal and cognitive difficulties such as delayed language development, with motor coordination and auditory processing issues. IQ levels are 20 points below controls, and verbal IQ

is the lowest of the four IQ levels[13]
- Performs best in stable families, but struggles with self-esteem and stress-management issues
- Tall, with accelerated growth until puberty
- Trouble forming stable interpersonal relationships
- Most have no signs and symptoms

C. Origins

- SRY is missing or is present on the X chromosome
- The child's mother is typically past age 35

D. Background

- Most do not know they have a chromosomal difference
- Is not rare since it affects 1 in 1,000 female births but often goes undetected[13]
- Reared as a girl

E. Therapeutic Interventions

- Perform Standard Sexual Assessment (Appendix C), medical assessment, and obtain a sexual and medical history from the girl's parents, especially

contributing factors
- Assess early and involve pediatric geneticist, psychologist, and teachers
- Obtain EEG and MRI
- Implement early speech therapy, physiotherapist, psychological, behavioral, and educational support as need arises
- Initiate hormone therapy
- Early elective genital surgery not indicated

F. Supportive Interventions

- Review the Supportive Interventions Guide for Children (Appendix G)
- Assist child with stress-management techniques
- Administer psychotropic medications if psychoses present
- Promote and encourage positive self-esteem activities
- Use calming techniques to manage child's labile emotions
- Assist the child with learning difficulties and obtain expert interventions as needed

G. Potential Outcomes

- Does best in a stable family and usually experience overall improvement when become adults
- Are mostly fertile, do have children, and do well parenting
- Some medical professionals do not regard Triple X as a disability
- Most can function in society and lead healthy, productive lives

4. Sexual Developmental Incongruence in Children Due to a Hormonal Variance

These include a) complete androgen insensitivity, b) partial androgen insensitivity, and c) mild androgen insensitivity

4a) Complete Androgen Insensitivity (cAIS)

A. Definition. cAIS is a condition that affects the sexual development of a child before birth and during puberty. The child is genetically male (one X and one Y chromosome), but is resistant to androgen (male hormones). As a result, the person has some or all the physical traits of a woman but the genetic makeup of a man."[14(p1)]

B. Signs and Symptoms

- Genetically male, but genitals may appear to be female or somewhere in between due to under-masculinization; has male or female characteristics
- The child develops testes during gestation that produce Mullerian Inhibiting hormone, so Mullerian structure (epididymis, vas deferens, seminal vesicles) are absent; 50% have hernias that usually contain testes[14]
- No spermatogenesis and lacks uterus, fallopian tubes, cervix, and upper part of vagina[14]
- Has undescended or partially descended testes, with small penis or an enlarged clitoris
- Male chromosomes but female external appearance and female gender identity
- Reduced breast tissue, no uterus so no menses, and is infertile; no pubic or axillary hair at puberty[14]
- Child is often unaware has the condition
- Genitoplasty for cosmetic reasons is strongly resisted by many people with cAIS, sexologists, and other HCPs. If surgery is performed early, the sex of assignment must be determined by how the individual will live after puberty when becomes sexually active

C. Origins

- XY chromosome present, but a deficiency in the cells in the child's body renders the cells unable to respond to/metabolize available androgens[14]
- A change in the gene that produces androgen receptors

D. Background

- Affects 1 in 20,000 live births[14]
- Reared as girls

E. Therapeutic Interventions

- Perform a Standard Sexual Assessment (Appendix C) and a medical assessment, and obtain a sexual and medical history from the parents, especially history of contributing factors
- Refer to a pediatric endocrinologist, a geneticist, psychologist, pediatric general surgeon, and a family nurse practitioner (FNP). An FNP is a registered nurse who has completed and demonstrated competency in an advanced direct patient care role, with an emphasis on family practice. In some instances, a genital

reconstruction surgeon may also be needed
- Genetic counseling, pelvic ultrasound, levels of luteinizing hormone, and testosterone
- Child may not need personal counseling; parents mostly do
- Obtain pelvic ultrasound to determine the presence of testes
- Gradual, gentle vaginal dilatation and perhaps genitoplasty (restructure) surgery at a later date
- Estrogen hormone replacement therapy after puberty
- Removal of testes when growth complete

F. Supportive Interventions

- Review the Supportive Interventions Guide for Children (Appendix G)
- Ensure child told about condition before she reaches puberty
- Evaluate child and parents' level of understanding of condition and teach accordingly
- Provide emotional support to parents, and reinforce psychological expert interventions
- Encourage parents to explain the process of puberty to the child and reinforce
- Explain the rationale for hormone replacement,

teach how to administer hormones, and check for medication compliance
- Educate about all other medications and treatment protocols
- Encourage a discussion of child's body image and promote positive self-image
- Pre- and post-operative care if has a hernia with testes corrected
- Observe for any psychological issues

G. Potential Outcomes

- Testes in pelvis may need removal as may become malignant
- Most often describes self as female; adds heterosexual to description as matures; many have orgasms
- Infertile, but some may become mothers through adoption
- Lifespan not usually shortened, but may have psychological and social concerns

4b) Partial Androgen Insensitivity (pAIS)

A. Definition. pAIS is a condition in which there is partial sensitivity to androgen in the child's cells that results in a genetically male baby with various levels of genital ambiguity. A child with a high level of insensitivity will develop as a girl during puberty, while a child with a low level of insensitivity will develop as a boy; the level of sensitivity determines how genitals develop

B. Signs and Symptoms

- Condition of pAIS usually determined at birth
- The child has a predominantly male-looking body with female, male, or both sex characteristics, and a male or female gender identity
- Clitoris may be larger than usual and penis small, or vice versa, with or without hypospadias present
- May be raised as a boy or girl

C. Origins

- As with complete androgen insensitivity, but has some androgen sensitivity

D. Background Information

- Brought up either as a girl or boy, and usually retains the sex assigned at birth

- Incidence same as for cAIS; 1 in 20,000 live births

E. Therapeutic Interventions

- Perform a Standard Sexual Assessment (Appendix C) and medical assessment, and obtain a sexual and medical history from parents, especially history of contributing factors
- Refer to a pediatric endocrinologist, geneticist, psychologist, FNP, pediatric surgeon
- Genetic counseling, pelvic ultrasound, levels of luteinizing hormone and testosterone
- Hernia repair and testes removal
- Girls who have had testes removed will need estrogen replacement for menopausal symptoms and osteoporosis
- Boys will need testosterone and perhaps delayed puberty hormones
- Genital surgery for genitoplasty at an early age is controversial; no immediate elective genital surgery at birth indicated
- Ensure child told of pAIS condition before puberty

"Perform no major surgery for cosmetic reasons alone; only for conditions related to physical/mental health.

This will entail a great deal of explanation needed for the parents who will want their children to 'look normal.' Explain to them that appearances during childhood, while not typical of other children, may be of less importance than functionality and post erotic sensitivity of the genitalia. Surgery can potentially impair sexual/erotic function. Therefore such surgery, which includes all clitoral surgery and any sex reassignment, should typically wait until puberty or after when the patient is able to give truly informed consent."

— Milton Diamond

F. Supportive Interventions

- Review the Supportive Interventions Guide for Children (Appendix G)
- Reinforce genetic counseling before puberty
- Explain usual childhood sexual development to the child, and why the child has a genital variance
- Explain to boys why they need androgens at puberty for male characteristics, and to girls why they need estrogens to prevent menopausal symptoms
- Be forthright and answer all questions about sexuality, fertility, delayed puberty, and secondary sex characteristics directly

- Educate about all medications and treatment protocols; check for compliance

G. Potential Outcomes

- Most people lead normal, productive lives, albeit with some psychological, interpersonal, and social issues
- Usual life expectancy
- All girls will be infertile, as will most boys

4c) Mild Androgen Insensitivity (mAIS)

A. Definition. Similar to pAIS but with less insensitivity

B. Signs and Symptoms

- Male-looking body with male genitalia, so the child may never know he has this condition

C. Origins

- Same as cAIS and pAIS

D. Background

- Occurs less frequently than cAIS and pAIS
- Reared as boys

E. Therapeutic Interventions

- Perform Standard Sexual Assessment (Appendix C) and medical assessment, and obtain a sexual and medical history from parents, especially history of contributing factors
- Refer to a general surgeon to reduce breasts if indicated
- Ongoing observation, with limited frequency as the child gets older
- Determine whether needs hormone support
- Breast reduction for the boy may or may not be indicated after puberty

F. Supportive Interventions

- Review the Supportive Interventions Guide for Children (Appendix G)
- The need for education about mAIS and any ramifications for the child are usually minimal

G. Potential Outcomes

- Boys lead healthy, productive lives, and most have

no awareness of their condition
- Often infertile, with breast enlargement at puberty

5a) Hypospadias

A. Definition. A congenital condition in which a boy's urethral opening does not form at the tip of the penis; instead, it is located somewhere along the penile shaft. May result in a penis that not only looks different but may also perform inefficiently

B. Signs and Symptoms

- At birth, a boy's urethral opening may not be located as usual at the tip of the boy's penis; instead, it may be located at any point along the underside of the penis, including the base of the penis. This results in a spray of urine instead of a steady stream
- The boy may also have a curved penis (15%), with incompletely developed foreskin[15]
- In 8% of boys with hypospadias, one testicle may not be fully descended. A small percentage of infant boys may have no testicles at all[15]

C. Origins

Cause is unknown, but hormonal variances occur between 9 and 12 weeks of life in utero when male hormones usually form the urinary channel and foreskin. A variance in the process during this period may be implicated in hypospadias

D. Background

- Hypospadias is a congenital variance that affects 4 in 1000 boys[15]
- Of boys with hypospadias, 7% have a father who has hypospadias also, the second son has a 12% chance of hypospadias, and if brother and father are affected, the possibility goes up to 21%[15]
- Reared as boys

E. Therapeutic Interventions

- Perform a Standard Sexual Assessment (Appendix C) and medical assessment and obtain a sexual history from parents, especially history of contributing factors
- Penile surgery (to straighten shaft, create urinary

canal, position urethral opening at penile head, and foreskin reconstruction) is indicated between ages 3–18 months to prevent problems such as difficulty with urination and/or maintaining an erection later in life[15]

F. Supportive Interventions

- Review the Supportive Interventions Guide for Children (Appendix G)
- Provide education to child and parents regarding preoperative care for general anesthesia and post-operative care
- Provide pain management, infection prevention management, catheter care, skin and wound care, urinary elimination/observation, and child and parent reassurance
- Give parents support and inform parents about anticipated outcomes
- Educate parents about the condition, post-operative home care, and follow-up visits

G. Potential Outcomes

- Most conditions of hypospadias are resolved with

Unexpected Sexual Behaviors

one surgery; the remainder, except for a very small minority, resolve with the second repair
- The most common complication of this corrective surgery is the formation of a fistula
- Boys usually have no memory of surgery, and there are usually no gender issues

6. Cryptorchidism (Hidden or Undescended Testes) in Boys

    A. Definition. An undescended testicle (cryptorchidism or *hidden testicle*) is a condition in which a testicle has not moved into its proper position in the bag of the scrotum before a boy's birth. Usually, one testicle is affected, but about 10% of the time, both testicles are involved[16]

    B. Signs and Symptoms

- Absence of a testicle in the scrotal sac (where usually expected to be)
- Testes palpable in the lower abdomen, or detected via ultrasound

    C. Origins

- No known cause, although the health and habits of the mother (smoking, diabetes, obesity), maternal hormones, environmental factors, among others may contribute

D. Background

- Hypspadias is the most common male congenital, genital anomaly in that it affects 3% of full-term male infants and up to 30% of premature male infants[17]
- In most cases, the undeveloped testicle descends into its correct place within the first few months of life. The testicle may move back and forth from the sac into the lower abdomen unassisted. Often associated with the presence of hypospadias
- Within the first year of life, 70% of affected testicles spontaneously descend, but approximately 1% of boys with undescended testicles still have testicles in the abdomen[17]

E. Therapeutic Interventions

- Perform a Standard Sexual Assessment (Appendix C) and medical assessment, and obtain a sexual and medical history from parents, especially history of contributing factors

Unexpected Sexual Behaviors

- Evaluate hormonal status and implement human chorionic gonadotropin to determine whether testicular tissue remains. A rise in the testosterone levels indicates that viable testicular tissue is present.[17] If testosterone is not elevated, there is no need for laparoscopy or abdominal surgery. Ultrasound, MRI, CT scans may be performed
- Prescribe androgens to promote testicular descent
- Assess the child's lower abdomen to determine whether surgery/laparoscopy is appropriate; perform while under one year in order to have fewer complications later
- May be treated medically with hormones
- Locate the testicle during surgery, and if vessel is adequate, insert and suture into the scrotal sac. Determine whether other approaches are possible after vessel elongates with time. If a hernia is present, that is also repaired
- Clinical uncertainty and lack of guidance exist on the appropriate clinical pathway for the treatment of cryptorchidism[17]
- Orchidectomy (removal of the testicle) may need to be performed if the testicle is not viable

F. Supportive Interventions

- Review the Supportive Interventions Guide for Children (Appendix G)
- Explain the intended plan of care to the parents and reassure the young boy
- Administer hormones to raise androgen levels, and observe boy for descended testicles
- Prepare the child for surgery, and administer preoperative medications
- Provide post-operative care to observe for nausea, bleeding, torsion, anxiety, and nausea

G. Potential Outcomes

- There may be complications such as malignancy (an untreated undescended testicle may become malignant), infertility, or strangulation of the spermatic cord
- Surgery mostly results in a cure, except if the testicle is too poorly developed to preserve
- Successful repair usually promotes a positive self-esteem in the boy and prevention of testicular malignancy in later life

Points for Discussion:

Ask yourself: Should physicians perform sex assignment surgery on infants with ambiguous genitalia soon after birth or delay until the child's sexual maturity? Please provide your rationale.

Ask yourself: Should physicians delay puberty on children until they can make a more informed decision, or should they let *nature* run its natural course? Please provide your rationale.

7. Congenital Adrenal Hyperplasia

A. Definition. Congenital adrenal hyperplasia (CAH) encompasses a group of autosomal recessive disorders, each of which involves a deficiency of an enzyme involved in the synthesis of cortisone, aldosterone, or both. A deficiency of 21 hydroxylase is the most common form of CAH, accounting for over 90% of cases.[18]

B. Signs and Symptoms

- Some infants with CAH may be born with typical female internal and external genitalia, or a large clitoris that resembles a penis or fused labia that resemble testes
- Boys will appear normal at birth even if they have a severe form of the disease, but precocious sexual and

body changes may occur in boys as early as age nine. Boys may be taller, with an adult body build, pubic hair, and a larger than usual penis for age; sometimes they may engage in inappropriate sexual behavior usually associated with increased libido[19]
- Girls may show signs of precocious puberty as early as six to eight years, especially African-American girls, with early pubic and axillary hair growth and breasts. Girls with a milder form of CAH may have no signs and symptoms until they reach puberty, and they may have ovaries, uterus, and fallopian tubes. Girls with the severe form of CAH usually have variant genitalia at birth
- May be present in boys as well as girls, and affects 1 in 10,000 to 20,000 babies[19]
- Genetic female masculinized as masculinization process continues after birth; boyish, with a deep, masculine voice as a child
- Girls have a failure to menstruate but feel strongly that they are girls
- They are tall children, but become small adults
- Most are reared as girls and mostly have 46,XX phenotype but this can vary

C. Origins

- Usually the adrenal glands produce hormones such as cortisol (maintains blood pressure and adrenal androgens), and the adrenal androgens also influence secondary sex characteristics. This leads to an androgen excess and a cortisol deficit and results in an XX chromosome female baby[20]
- Speiser[20] states that a 21-hydroxylase deficiency (most common at 95% of occurrences) causes a miscommunication in typical cortisol synthesis
- The above leads to an androgen excess and a cortisol deficit, which results in an XX female baby with a large clitoris and male-like appearance, excessive hair, and precocious behavior[21]

D. Background

- The child requires healthcare observations throughout life for maintenance of cortisol, aldosterone, and electrolytes
- Mostly reared as girls

E. Therapeutic Interventions

E$_1$. Initial Therapeutic Interventions

- Perform a Standard Sexual Assessment (Appendix C) and medical assessment, and obtain a sexual and medical history from parents, especially history of contributing factors and mother's obstetrical history
- Confirm CAH through administration of a test dose of synthetic CAH,[22] and obtain other needed blood levels
- Obtain x-ray of left hand (usually larger in a child with CAH)
- Perform newborn screening (Newborn screening for a number of diseases, including CAH, 21-hydroxylase, glucocorticoid, and mineral corticoid levels is done in all 50 states)[22]
- The salt-losing form of CAH threatens the life of the infant, so rapidly treat the infant with cortisol, aldosterone, glucose, potassium, and sodium to maintain hormones and electrolytes to reach as normal a level as possible[21]
- The use of emergency genitoplasty to "correct" the genitals of a newborn infant with CAH requires great thought and discussion between parents, physicians, and a psychologist, among others

- Discuss with peers the perceived natal sex of the child after a review of all the available information; do not decide hastily as no medical emergency exists to "fix" genitals
- While genetic tests help diagnose or confirm the decision, they cannot change them. Most babies are female, but that is not always the case
- Inform parents of the child's sexual ambiguity, support them, and actively involve them in the decision-making process

E$_2$. Maintenance Therapeutic Interventions

- Monitor baby regularly for all potential areas of concern, to include blood pressure, blood glucose and aldosterone levels, and electrolytes
- Special attention to a baby is required around three weeks of age when the severest form of the disease presents itself
- Continue hormone replacement with oral glucocorticoids, e.g., cortisol, hydrocortisone, and aldosterone replacement as needed
- Maintain family and child support with timely sharing of all results
- Educate parents about the potential for serious crises if electrolytes are severely abnormal

- Educate parents about the expected outcomes of the child's condition
- Arrange for community and discharge support for child and parents
- Develop a team approach to include a pediatric and medical endocrinologist, urologist, surgeon, a geneticist, psychologist, and pediatric nurses experienced in care of children with CAH
- Continue medical management throughout child's life, especially hormones and electrolytes, especially during puberty
- Testes may be removed if present due to malignancy potential
- Implement medications for excessive virilization management
- Genetic counseling and psychological counseling for parents; child may not need counseling since the condition is all that he or she knows

"The incredible lesson about our sexual biology is that all men at one point in their fetal development have the capacity to be a woman. Moreover the body is programmed to develop as female unless it sees and recognizes specific biochemical signals such as

testosterone and anti-mullerian factor that tell it to develop as male."

— *Abraham Morgentaler*
(in reference to cases of testicular feminization)

F. Supportive Interventions

F₁. Initial Supportive Interventions

- Review the Supportive Interventions Guide for Children (Appendix C)
- During the early days of baby's life monitor her vital signs, fluids, and electrolytes diligently as the severe electrolyte imbalance can occur rapidly with the life-threatening consequences of Cushing's disease (increase in cortisol levels) and Addison's disease (decrease in cortisone and aldosterone levels)[18]
- Administer sodium chloride rapidly, followed by long-term glucocorticoids and mineral corticoids to suppress androgen production. Administer aldosterone replacement and sodium intravenously. Add sodium chloride to infant's formula, and always have injectable mineral/glucocorticoids available[18]
- Provide parents with education, both written and verbal, regarding genital and bodily ambiguity and the

- expected immediate condition process
- Answer questions when requested about potential overall outcomes, but avoid being drawn into discussions with the family about the biological sex of the infant; isolated opinions are not only inappropriate, but they confuse the parents
- Provide emotional and practical support to parents
- Arrange for social services and perhaps a spiritual adviser

F_2. Maintenance Supportive Interventions

- Observe infant for cardiac arrythmias, poor feeding, vomiting, diarrhea, weight loss, and salt wasting, which occurs most often when a baby is about three weeks old
- Instruct parents that treatment will continue for life; the reasons for use of the emergency kit, contents of the kit, and use of the emergency kit; how to give injections of cortisone and other medications, and why, when and how to summon help
- Prepare parents at the appropriate time for their child's potential development and behavior during the toddler years, early childhood, and puberty
- Support the counseling of parents about how to raise their child in the determined natal sex: male, female,

Unexpected Sexual Behaviors

or (rarely) gender neutral, and prepare them for anticipated changes
- Teach parents to observe for signs of early maturation, for excessive hair growth, especially pubic and armpit hair, body odor, and early sexual maturity
- Administer medications to slow skeletal maturation and decrease virilization
- Evaluate the potential for precocious behavior and genital appearance, and respond to questions about topics such as sexual maturity, early puberty, puberty-suppressing medications, among others
- Provide ongoing education about the child's condition, growth, puberty, and expectations
- Counsel parents about the seriousness if a fever, stress, an illness, vomiting, or diarrhea occur, and the need to increase dose of cortisol during stress; never miss a cortisol dose. Teach that the child must always wear a medical alert identification

G. Potential Outcomes

- "75% of classic CAH suffer episodes of aldosterone deficiency, with salt-wasting, failure to thrive, and potentially fatal hypovolemia and shock"[21(p2)]
- Male babies may be misdiagnosed and may die because

- they have no apparent genital variance
- Children with CAH must take medications for the remainder of their lives
- Most have happy, productive lives; however, they are always aware of their condition, the potential for life-threatening episodes, and the need to maintain healthcare follow-up
- Gender issues may or may not be a great concern as most feel and act like women
- Emergency genitoplasty may be performed on the baby when there is no indication to do so. Emergency genitoplasty is **not supported** by persons with adult CAH or sexologists[23]

8. Child Sexual Abuse

"Children who are victimized through sexual abuse often begin to develop deeply held tenets that shape their concept of self: 'My worth is my sexuality. I'm dirty and shameful. I have no right to my own physical boundaries.' That shapes their ideas about the world around them: 'No one will believe me. Telling the truth results in bad consequences. People can't be trusted.' It doesn't take long for children to begin to act in accordance with these belief systems. For girls who have experienced incest, sexual abuse or rape, the boundaries between love, sex, and pain become blurred. Secrets are normal, and shame is a constant."

— Rachel Lloyd, Sexual Activist

"When asked to describe their most difficult patient condition to care for, many HCPs place child abuse cases at the very top of their list. Most of us can deal (intellectually, at least) with the ravages of cancer or the deterioration that comes with aging, child mistreatment can be much harder to cope with emotionally."[24 (p1, para1)] "The first step toward helping a child who may have been a victim of child sex abuse (CSA) is to understand how sexual abuse is defined, behaviors that may indicate abuse has occurred, how those behaviors may differ from typical sexual behaviors in children, and how sexual abuse may affect children."[25 (p1, para1)]

A. **Definition.** According to the American Psychological Association,[26] there is no universal definition for CSA. In operative terms, it is the coercion by an adult of a child, followed by sexual contact activities such as touching the child's genitals and masturbation, oral-genital contact, finger penetration of vagina and/or anus, and less-frequently, vaginal and anal intercourse. Non-contact CSA includes body exposure, voyeurism, and child pornography.

B. **Signs and Symptoms**

- Children and adolescents may present with a range of psychological and behavioral problems, from mild to severe, both short and long term. Some of these

include depression, anxiety, guilt, eating disorders, sleep problems, and withdrawal
- Younger age behaviors such as thumb-sucking, bedwetting, eating problems, sleep problems, and school and social problems occur
- The strongest indication of child sexual abuse is inappropriate sexual knowledge and interest in sexual behavior. In addition, the child may present with evidence of sexually transmitted diseases (STIs) and pain[26]

C. Origins

- Perpetrator was exposed to domestic violence during childhood and/or experienced personal emotional and physical neglect
- A frequently heard statement is that 95% of offenders are known to the child and 5% are strangers
- The offender may have been sexually abused as a child
- The perpetrator selects a known child as a victim (rarely a stranger), to whom the offender has easy access; grooming of the child then takes place. Initially, a non-sexual relationship takes place, and the offender becomes a *special* friend to the child. Eventually, the offender introduces sexual activities into the relationship[27]

D. Background

- The World Health Organization (WHO)[28(p1)] estimates that more than 800 million worldwide may have experienced CSA, with more than 500 million having experienced contact or intercourse types of abuse; "more than is comfortable or plausible"
- The precise incidence of CSA is unknown and underreported due to the child's fears of retaliation from the offender, self-shame, and self-blame, fear and embarrassment, as well as a lack of consensus about definition, and inadequate tracking[29]
- Homosexual men are no more likely to abuse children than heterosexual men, and women sexually abuse children less frequently than men
- Most children who have sexual activities with an adult have just one interaction, or if more than one interaction, it is with the same person[29]
- "12 percent of men and 17 percent of women reported that they had been touched sexually when they were children. As girls they were touched most often by family adult males, less often by adolescent males; while the boys were touched more often by adolescent girls, less often by adolescent boys, and even less by an adult male"[29(p380)]

- Most of the adult to child contacts involve the adult touching the child's genitals; oral contacts and vaginal and anal penile penetration occur less frequently
- About one third of children are under the age of seven when the sexual contact with a male occurs and two-thirds between ages 7-10 years. The difference in age between girls as the victims and adolescent boys as the offenders is usually just a few years[29]
- According to APA[26] there is no difference in incidences of CSA regardless of race, culture, or economic status; however:
- Brown and Finkelhorn[30] reported that the sexual abuse is inverse to socioeconomic status
- Most sexually abused children are female
- Investigating allegations of sexual abuse of children is very difficult for law enforcement personnel. Resolution of these cases is frequently hindered by victim reluctance to talk about the incident due to shame, embarrassment, etc., or an inability to communicate, as well as a scarcity of corroborating evidence[31]
- In all 50 states, medical personnel, mental health professionals, teachers, and law enforcement personnel are required by law to report suspected abuse, even if not validated at the time. Reporting CSA is an instance where the nurse does not violate HIPAA expectations

if he or she reports an incident

E. Therapeutic Interventions

- Centers for CSA treatment usually have a multidisciplinary team that includes a physician or a psychologist, a forensic nurse, a pediatric nurse practitioner, and a social worker, all experienced in the management of CSA
- Obtain history from parents without the child present, especially history of contributing factors, but when interview the child if over age three, ask the parents to wait outside[32]
- Examine the child's behavior carefully. The physician must diligently differentiate between what are expected and developmentally appropriate sexual behaviors and what are sexual behavior problems in the child
- Head-to-toe exam to include observation for bleeding, bruises, fractures (old and new), pain, (include mouth), discharge, burns, and an anal-genital examination for bruising, bleeding, trauma, lacerations, scarring, anal dilation
- Obtain specimens such as a throat culture, blood or lesion scraping for STIs, photographs, and perhaps trace forensic evidence collection
- Assess for signs of physical abuse, other illnesses, and

pregnancy
- Assess the child to determine how he or she functions with stressors, past and present
- Assess the child's emotional state, coping strategies such as acting out with anger or sadness, the child's friendships, strengths, communication skills, and the attachments to adults in the child's life
- Determine what type of therapy would benefit the child, individual, group, or family: **Individual therapy** includes music, art, talk, and play or combinations. **Group therapy** involves the child meeting in groups with other children who have also been sexually abused to learn new skills through role play, discussion, games, and play. **Family therapy** involves the child and parents meeting with therapists to improve communication and to help the parents learn new skills that help the child behave appropriately

F. Supportive Interventions

F$_1$. Initial Supportive Interventions

- Review the Supportive Interventions Guide for Children (Appendix G)
- Examine the child's behavior carefully. The FNP or

forensic nurse expert must accurately differentiate between what are reasonable and developmentally appropriate sexual behaviors and what are sexual behavior problems in the child
- Forensic nurse expert to explain his/her role and planned interventions in a language the child and parents understand. If the child is over age three, talk to the child without the parents present[32]
- Initiate and administer all prescribed medications, with explanations to parents and child
- Ensure the child is comfortable and has all physical and emotional needs met (as much as within reason)
- Monitor child that all her vital signs are within normal limits
- Refer to facility social services department and Department of Children and Family Services, as needed

F_2. Child Advocacy Interventions
- The most important role of the HCP is to be the child's advocate to maintain the child's health and safety, not to prove the existence of child sexual abuse or to treat the child psychologically
- Maintain a safe environment within the facility for the child before, during, and after nursing care has been provided

- Collaborate with the physician, forensic nurse specialist, FNP or other nurses, and other healthcare professionals to assure adherence to all facility, state, and legal expectations—especially the notification and documentation of findings to facilitate appropriate child placement and legal compliance

F_3. Child Education Interventions

Teach the child and caregivers that:
- A child's body belongs only to the child; nobody else may touch a child's private parts
- The child should have no secrets; must never go off anywhere with a stranger; should always be with a known person, including going to the bathroom, and never go off alone
- Children should never be urged or cajoled to hug or kiss an adult or family friend; they should do so spontaneously and of their own volition
- If a child sees a stranger, most often a man, waiting around the playground at school or in the park, she is to tell an adult she knows
- Caregivers must always know the child's playmates
- Caregivers are to demonstrate cautious behaviors around the child, but minimize use of scare tactics

Unexpected Sexual Behaviors

- Actively listen and believe what the child states; validate later
- Provide a safe place, free of distraction and child-friendly; let the child choose her own place to sit and maintain her comfort distance. Ensure the child's privacy, but do not leave a child alone
- Introduce self calmly, softly, and interact confidently and non-threateningly with the child
- Avoid excessive hugging, touching, etc., as this might confuse the child. Ask the child her name and what name she prefers. Tell her where she is, and if she is young, explain in understandable terms why you are there

F_4. Maintenance Supportive Interventions

- Review the Supportive Interventions Guide for Children (Appendix G)
- Ask as few questions as possible, and avoid leading questions
- Ask the child to talk about herself when she is comfortable to do so and reassure her that she has done nothing wrong
- If care providers have been informed and are available, encourage them to remain calm and in control; the greater the alarm and distress of caregivers, the greater

the child's residual trauma
- Never hurry the child, nor be impatient, and convey your support without excess emotion
- When the child talks, listen and let her describe how she felt during the sexual activity; allow her to tell her story in her own time and manner. Use crayons, pencils, paper, and other devices through which the child might want to depict her feelings. Mental health professionals only use anatomically correct dolls in *play scenarios*
- Convey to the child that she did not deserve the abuse, and she is not responsible for the actions of the offending adult

G. Potential Outcomes

- Most sexually abused children lead productive lives and do not become sex abusers themselves. However, "Factors that seem to affect the amount of harm done include the age of the child, the duration, the frequency, and intrusiveness of the abuse; the degree of force used, and the relationship of the abuser to the child"[26 (p1,para11)]
- When a child or adolescent is not believed by people he or she trusts when reporting the CSA, he or she may suffer a range of psychological and behavioral problems. These include depression, anxiety, guilt, and

withdrawal, and regression behaviors such as thumb-sucking, bedwetting, eating problems, sleep problems, and school and social problems
- The strongest indication of CSA is inappropriate sexual knowledge and interest in and actual sexual behavior by the child. If a child is reassured that she bears no guilt, the potential damage to the child is reduced; similarly, if the response by parents/caregivers is not overly emotional or widespread, the damage is lessened. Family support, extra-familial support, high self-esteem, and spirituality are helpful to prevent symptoms as adults, as well as the relinquishment of guilt and the passage of time[26]

9. Harmful Sexual Behavior (or Sexual Behavior Problems) in Children

The term *sexual* is often used to describe certain behaviors of children, but these behaviors are rarely related to sexual self-gratification or self-stimulation. Instead, these behaviors are related to other factors such as childhood curiosity, impulsivity, anxiety, trauma attributed to PTSD, and attention-seeking activities[33]

A. Definition. Harmful sexual behavior or sexual behavior problems (SBP) that involve one or more children engaging in sexual discussions or acts that are inappropriate for their age or stage of development. These can range from using sexually explicit words and phrases to full penetrative sex with other children[34]

B. Signs and Symptoms

- The **sexually inappropriate** child makes sexual remarks, gestures, touches, or exposes own genitals, or similar behaviors, but with no contact with another child[35]
- The **sexually intrusive** child grabs another child's genitals; then he runs away, or he rubs against another person in a sexually provocative manner, or he briefly fondles another person, but stops when the other person is angry or upset[35]
- The **sexually aggressive** child is coercive or aggressive in his sexual behavior; there is significant or prolonged contact resulting in completion of a sexual act such as oral sex, vaginal or anal penetration, mutual masturbation, or similar behaviors[35]

C. Origins

- A history of offender sexual abuse as well as the powerlessness that the abused felt during that abuse may contribute
- Increased exposure to sexually explicit material at a younger age; stress, especially parental divorce; deficits in social skills and social competence;[34] peer pressure; lack of timely parental intervention; neglect; lack of self-control; violence in the home; inadequate rules regarding privacy and boundaries; and a culture that punishes sexual behavior
- The schizophrenic-like attitudes toward sex in today's Western society that lead to a child's skewed impression of what appropriate sexual behavior is

D. Background

- These children come from all socioeconomic levels, but there is over-representation of children from lower socioeconomic levels
- Rich[34] found that there is cause for concern if there is an age difference of two years or more, or if one child is pre-pubertal and one post-pubertal
- Harmful sexual behavior is not perceived as being

wrong when a child sees his peers doing it also
- Unacceptable sexual behavior by a child is often the result of damaged relationships, especially those critical to the child
- Results from standard psychological instruments revealed that children with sexual behavioral problems are more disturbed and pathological, especially those who demonstrate inappropriate and aggressive sexual behavior[35 (para2)]
- The link between CSA and child sexual behavior problems is well established
- "Mothers who are more educated and who acknowledge that sexual behaviors in children can be normal behaviors tend to report more sexual behaviors in their children when compared to mothers with fewer years of education and less acceptance of these behaviors"[36 (p1)]

E. Therapeutic Interventions
- Review the Supportive Interventions Guide for Children (Appendix G)
- Obtain physical and maturational history
- Obtain early psychological consultation for the child
- Differentiate between normative sexual activities of the child and pathological sexual activities that are often misdiagnosed and mislabeled
- Assess the child and his/her sexual behaviors: self-

directed or directed to others, coercive, and aggressive, with associated depression, among other issues
- Know that "Children with SBP are at a very low risk to commit future sex offenses if provided appropriate treatment"[37 (p200)]
- Assess caregivers' capacity, warmth and support, home environment, family relationships, boundaries, decision-making skills, and home discipline
- Determine and implement the most appropriate intervention from below:
    a. Cognitive Behavioral Therapy (CBT) is possibly the most beneficial approach because it changes the child's unwanted thinking patterns, and in so doing, changes unwanted behaviors
    b. According to Smallbone[38], The Multisystemic Therapy (MST) uses outcome-focused interventions for directly altering harmful or negative relationships
    c. 12 outpatient, one-hour group sessions for the children, as well as twelve, one-hour group sessions for parents or caregivers. The intent of the intervention is to reduce sexual behavior problems, to increase self-esteem, and improve parent-child relationships[35]
    d. One-on-one meetings with a mental health professional and the child alone, with the caregivers

and the child, with caregivers alone, and with persons with whom the child has relationships, especially a child's peers

- Determine whether the child has any psychological issues such as depression, suicidal thoughts, aggressive/coercive behaviors, etc., and if so, carefully determine what future placement may be needed—home, inpatient, outpatient, residential care, state facility, or foster home
- Use medications sparingly and mostly for the sexually aggressive child
- Other interventions such as the use of reading, storytelling, drawing, videos, etc., have some effect

F. Supportive Interventions

- Review the Supportive Interventions Guide for Children (Appendix G)
- Know and differentiate between standard sexual themes of the child and pathological ones
- Use a one-on-one with the child or CBT with a peer group approach or a CBT with a child and parent approach to the discussion of issues and evaluate the effectiveness

- Assess child for excessive nudity and masturbation, inappropriate sexual touching of others, sexual language, and other sexual behaviors
- Teach the caregivers to establish ground rules for the child to include spatial and physical boundaries, privacy, curfews, nudity, etc.
- Teach the caregiver how to provide child sex education at educational and age level of understanding
- Encourage and facilitate a private discussion with the child about previous episodes of inappropriate sexual behavior or CSA with a witness present
- Assess episodes of inappropriate sexual behavior compared to other events in the child's life for a correlation in activities
- Perform all other necessary procedures and observations for STIs, physical abuse, psychological issues, academic problems

G. Potential Outcomes

- Children with sexual behavioral problems are more disturbed and pathological, especially those who demonstrate inappropriate and aggressive sexual behavior[35]
- According to Rich,[34] children who receive adequate

treatments are less likely to commit abuse as adults compared to children who receive no support; 5% versus 14% to 30%
- Children with childhood sexual behavior problems respond well to treatment, especially if done with active parental or caregiver support and participation

10.   Female Genital Mutilation.

"Muslim groups describe the fight against female genital mutilation (FGM) as 'our jihad,' and say it is a practice that is 'bringing Islam into disrepute.'....It is the first time that the Islamic Shari Council, the Muslim College, and the Muslim Council of Great Britain have joined together to condemn FGM, which may affect 20,000 British girls. 'FGM is not an Islamic requirement. There is no reference in the Koran that girls must be circumcised.' 'FGM is an oppressive cultural practice that has no place in the civilised world. It has got nothing to do with religion and is not condoned by Islam.' 'All the moderate voices, the correct voices of Islam must come out. We need to take a stand.'"

— *The Times* (London, England, May 2014)

A. **Definition.** "Female genital mutilation or cutting (FGM/FGC), comprises all procedures that involve partial or total removal of the female genitalia or other injury to the genitals for non-medical reasons. FGM/FGC is recognized as a violation of the human rights of girls and women, and also violates the person's rights to health, security, and physical integrity, the right to be free from torture and cruel, inhuman or degrading treatment, and the right to life when the procedure results in death."[39 (p1,para5)]

(Note: use of the word *mutilation* has been discouraged by supporters of the practice and use of the word *cutting* encouraged as they feel mutilation indicates malice and demonizes the practice they support. Others who do not support the practice feel the word *mutilation* is appropriate.

B. **Signs and Symptoms**

- A girl, usually between birth and age 15 (sometimes during infancy but most often between ages 7 and 10), is subjected by adults to a partial or total removal of her genital organs
- The World Health Organization (WHO) has identified four types of FGM[39]:
  - **Type 1:** Excision of the prepuce, with or without excision of part or all of the clitoris

- **Type 2:** Excision of the clitoris with partial or total excision of the labia minora
- **Type 3:** Excision of part or all of the external genitalia and stitching and narrowing of the vaginal opening (infibulation). Sometimes referred to as pharaonic
- **Type 4:** Others, such as pricking, piercing, or incising; stretching, burning of the clitoris, scraping of tissue surrounding the vaginal orifice, cutting the vagina; introduction of corrosive substances or herbs into the vagina to cause bleeding or tighten the opening
- Elderly women *(excisers)*[39] mostly perform this procedure within the community for a fee, without anesthesia or aseptic techniques, sometimes with special knives, but often with glass, scalpels, or razor blades. Sometimes medical practitioners (18% are HCPs)[39] perform the procedure for a fee that gives cause for alarm, that educated people condone and practice this extreme violation

C. Origins

- Culturally influenced and determined by adults within various communities, predominantly those

communities of the Islamic faith, even though the practices are not officially sanctioned by Islam
- According to the United Nations Population Fund (UNFPA), 2014,[40] FGM is performed for numerous reasons, (mostly myths that perpetuate the practice) to include:
  - **Psychosexual reasons:** to control a woman's *insatiable* sexuality that might occur if the clitoris remains. It is performed to ensure virginity before marriage and fidelity after, and to increase the sexual pleasure of a man
  - **Sociological and cultural reasons:** seen as a girl's initiation into womanhood; an intrinsic part of the community's cultural heritage/tradition, to enhance fertility, to promote child survival
  - **Hygiene and esthetic reasons:** some communities regard women's external genitalia as being dirty and ugly, so it is removed
  - **Religious reasons:** FGM is not sanctioned by Islam nor Christianity; however, some religious scripts are used to justify the practice, and many believe it has the support of some religious leaders
  - **Socio-economic reasons:** considered to be a prerequisite for marriage, (women are mostly dependent upon men), as well as their right to inherit

D. Background

- The practice predates Christianity and Islam. It was practiced in early Roman and Egyptian times, as well as in Africa, Ethiopia, and the Philippines, among other cultures
- The practice is most common in the 29 countries of Africa, Asia, and the Middle East; and increasingly in Western immigrant communities in Europe, Australia, Canada, and the United States [40]
- From 100 to 140 million girls have undergone some form of genital mutilation and cutting; at least 3 million girls are at risk for the procedure each year[40]
- Some progress has been made to reduce the practice over the past 40 years, although the change is extremely slow in some areas

E. Therapeutic Interventions

- Perform a Standard Sexual Assessment (Appendix C) and medical assessment, and obtain a sexual and medical history
- Ethically and legally, the procedure must not be supported, condoned, or practiced by physicians
- Provide all necessary care for associated complications

Unexpected Sexual Behaviors

- Report all known episodes of the practice to the legal authorities
- Always be cognizant of the risk of HIV
- Support, implement, and educate regarding strategies for the reduction/elimination of FGM/FGC
- Seven approaches have been adopted toward a reduction in FGM/FGC, to include education about associated health risks, conversion of *excisers*, training of healthcare professionals as change agents, alternative rituals, community-led approaches, public statements, and the introduction/enforcement of legal ramifications to include imprisonment (six months to life) and large financial penalties[41]

F. Supportive Interventions

- Review the Supportive Interventions Guide for Children (Appendix G)
- Ethically and legally, the procedure must not be condoned or practiced by HCPs
- Provide all necessary care for associated complications
- Report all known episodes of the practice to the legal authorities
- Support, implement, and educate regarding strategies for the reduction, then elimination of FGM/FGC

157

G. Potential Outcomes

- Immediate complications include severe pain, shock, hemorrhage, tetanus or septicemia, and surrounding tissue injury. Recurrent bladder and urinary tract infections, cysts, infertility, and complications of childbirth[39]
- Other effects include anemia, incontinence, dyspareunia, sexual dysfunction, and severe scar formation, among others
- Infibulation (removal of the clitoris, part or all of the labia minora, and surrounding tissues) results in a barrier to intercourse and later, childbirth, so the procedure has to be reversed (de-infibulation) for these to take place. Excessive thrusting by the male during the first sexual intercourse can result in severe bleeding, scar rupture, and perineal tears. The girl's wounds are then re-sutured.
- The girl may show signs of emotional scarring as well as physical scarring such as behavioral disturbances, loss of trust in caregivers, anxiety, depression, and marital conflict
- The risk of HIV is extensive due to the absence of aseptic techniques and the use of poorly constructed or sterilized instruments
- As the girl gets older, she may or may not support the

practice. However, community pressure to continue the practice in her daughters is difficult to overcome, especially within male-dominated societies

11. Sexually Transmitted Infections in Children

A. Definition. Sexually transmitted infections (STIs) in children are diseases that are transmitted mostly by sexual activities, usually during child sexual abuse (CSA) by an adult, transferred accidentally, or during childbirth. These conditions primarily consist of infections such as chlamydia, human papilloma virus, bacterial vaginosis, and HIV, among others.

B. Signs and Symptoms

- "The majority of children who have been sexually abused will have no physical complaints related either to trauma or STD infection. In children, the isolation of a sexually transmitted organism may be the first indication that abuse has occurred"[42 (p1)]

C. Origins

- STIs are usually transmitted from the mother's vagina to the boy's penis, the girl's vulva, or the child's eyes

during childbirth; from a penis to the girl's vagina; or from the penis to the anus or the anus to the penis during a sexual assault by an adult or a child's peer
- STIs in children are rarely transferred via fomites[42]

D. Background

- Because sexual assault is a violent crime that affects children of all ages, including infants, infants may become infected with an STI as well as children[31]
- The incubation periods for STIs vary from a few days for gonorrhea to several months for syphilis, and other STIs some time in between
- Rectal or vaginal infection of a child with chlamydia may indicate CSA, but the child's mother could have transferred the organism perinatally
- Children at high risk for having an STI include those whose sibling, parent, or another adult in the home is infected, those who have been sexually assaulted, those with genital lesions and an anal or vaginal discharge, and those for whom evidence exists of oral, vaginal, and/or anal penetration
- Other risk factors for STIs in children include a chaotic home, close relationship issues, unmet needs of the child, lack of emotional attachment, and physical and

emotional abuse
- STIs are extremely common in adolescents but not so in younger children as less chance exists for ascending infections. Chlamydia, gonorrhea, trichomonas, HPV (genital warts), herpes, and bacterial vaginitis are the most common STIs
- "STIs give rise to a range of anogenital and urinary tract diseases. The signs and symptoms of these diseases cluster into eight clinical syndromes. These include genital itching, genital ulcers, genital warts, urethritis, vaginal and cervical infections, epididymitis, pelvic inflammatory disease, and ano-rectal infections"[42 (p14)]

E. Therapeutic Interventions

- Perform a sexual assessment, but recognize that little information is usually obtained from the physical assessment; most is obtained from the parents, especially the history of contributing factors
- Minimize trauma and pain to the child at all points during examination and treatment, especially if the child has a vaginal discharge, existing pain, genital ulcers, itching, or urinary symptoms[43]
- Perform all diagnostic tests on the child before the start of any therapy

- Test for commonly occurring STIs (e.g., chlamydia) must be done before those that occur less frequently (e.g., syphilis)
- Perform visual inspection of vulva, penis, perineum, anus, and observe for discharge, odor, bleeding, irritation, warts, ulcerative lesions, and signs of trauma[43]
- Obtain swabs from the pharynx and anus of the boy or girl, vagina of the girl, and urethra of the boy, and test for all STIs. Repeat in one week where indicated
- Some STIs are required to be monitored and shared with government officials statewide and nationally; these include chancroid, chlamydia, gonorrhea, hepatitis A and B, HIV infections, and syphilis. However, frequently encountered STDs such as trichomoniasis, genital herpes, and HPV do not require government notification, even though they are at levels of concern in adults, and, therefore, a threat to children [42]
- Determine which organism is present and order appropriate medications,[42] to include:
    a) antibacterials to treat chancroid, chlamydia, gonorrhea, and syphilis
    b) antiretrovirals to treat genital herpes, genital warts, HIV, molluscum contagiosum
    c) antiprotozoals to treat trichomoniasis
    d) antiparasitics to treat pubic lice and scabies

e) vaccines to treat hepatitis
- "Because of the low prevalence of STIs in the prepubertal victims of sexual abuse, prophylactic therapy is not needed"[44 (p1,para8)]
- Involve an expert in HIV and AIDs care if positive results obtained, and determine whether prophylactic treatment for HIV is indicated. Perform HIV antibody testing at six weeks, three months, and six months[43]

F. Therapeutic Interventions

- Review the Supportive Interventions Guide for Children (Appendix G)
- HCPs must be experienced in the management of a child with an STI, or be mentored closely by one who is experienced
- Review referral data, to include location and STI infection, duration of infection, the incubation period, and potential sexual contacts
- Collaborate with the physician or FNP to determine the priority of the STI and plan the interventions needed
- Identify the risk factors for potential re-infection of the child for sexual abuse
- Encourage verbalization by the child and caregiver of feelings and expression of needs, to include safety and

- comfort needs, physical needs, emotional needs; and expression of fears, financial concerns, educational concerns, and school/peer/education concerns
- Implement actions toward resolution of those issues should they arise
- Obtain or assist the FNP or MD with specimen collection and specimen identification
- Monitor child that her vital signs are all within normal limits. Administer prescribed antibiotics, antivirals, vaccines, etc.
- If the presence of a positive STI is verified, inform the state registry of the incidence with associated details
- If CSA suspected, inform Department of Children and Family Services of findings
- Develop and implement safety measures, and if warranted, include suggestion to MD to order the removal of the child from his or her home
- Determine child's level of understanding of the STI and teach the child accordingly, using age and education appropriate levels
- Explain fully to the caregivers about the infection and the ramifications of non-compliance and lack of follow-up. Advise caregivers about medications, treatments, appointments, vaccinations, blood levels, and overall management of the STI involved

- Educate parents about potential for re-infection of the child if home situation or contact potential unchanged
- Explain the need for all family members to be checked and educated about STIs, or explain the potential for removal of the child

G. Potential Outcomes

- If the treatment protocol is continued and completed, the potential outcome for the child with an STI is usually excellent
- Issues arise when the child remains in a home environment where the threats of reinfection and CSA remain. Untreated, these STIs in the child may progress to a worse infection with sterility, ectopic pregnancy, pelvic inflammatory disease, malignancy, and other life-threatening diseases

CHAPTER 5

HIGH RISK SEXUAL BEHAVIORS BY AND AGAINST ADOLESCENTS AND THE CHALLENGES THESE BEHAVIORS PRESENT

"Most teens know plenty about the dangers of risk-taking behaviors like smoking, drinking, and taking drugs, but they are hardwired to ignore what they have learned. Teenagers seek out risk-taking behaviors because the brain systems involved in decision-making mature at different times."

— *Laurence Steinberg*

1. Sexual Coercion of American Adolescents

    A. Definition. "The act of using pressure, alcohol or drugs to have sexual contact with someone against his or her will;...tactics of post refusal persistence [used are] defined as persistent attempts to have sexual contact with someone who has already refused."[1]

B. Signs and Symptoms

- Evidence of emotional, physical, or verbal pressure by one person on another to make the victim participate in a sexual activity
- Actions used by the aggressor toward the victim are subtle as well as overt
- Victim often coerced into getting drunk to facilitate the sexual act

"I don't know what it is about men—not all men, but a good portion of them—that turned a good solid 'No' into an 'I'm just playing coy, try harder.'"

— Nenia Campbell

C. Origins

- Some feminist scholars feel that the origins of sexual coercion lie in the inequity that exists in sexual relationships, as well as the belief that violence is socially, not biologically, programmed[2]

- Alcohol excess, usually with binge-drinking and a history of casual sex, may make a potential victim an easy prey
- The majority of the time the victim has been a previous boyfriend or girlfriend, or a friend, or someone fairly well known to the victim

D. Background

- Sexual coercion exists in most age groups in America, but no more so than among adolescent college students who have just left high school and are exposed to a very different college life that may be exciting yet deceiving
- Sexual coercion occurs more frequently in the college lifestyle and environment, especially among younger, newer students among whom there are high levels of casual sexual activity
- Some view sexual coercion as less troublesome than some other sexual aggressive acts because of its persistent yet subtle emphasis. Coercion is a sexually aggressive act
- Often the victim has been in a relationship with the aggressor that ended against the aggressor's wishes

E. Therapeutic Interventions

- Perform a Standard Sexual Assessment (Appendix C) and medical assessment, and obtain a sexual and medical history
- Direct care therapeutic interventions are the same as for a post-rape situation
- Provide education about sexual coercion prevention, prevention of STDs, avoidance of binge-drinking of alcohol, avoidance of drugs, and use of campus risk management techniques to all new students, especially those just from high school
- Ensure all authorities notified according to law

F. Supportive Interventions

- Review the Supportive Interventions Guide for Adults (Appendix H)
- Encourage students to develop a close support system within the student body
- Promote methods to raise self-esteem of the student/victim, as well as sexual assertiveness techniques
- Encourage students to involve college authorities when incident first occurs, and not wait until repeated, as it most certainly will be

- Reinforce education about sexual coercion prevention, prevention of STDs, avoidance of binge-drinking of alcohol, avoidance of drugs, and use of campus risk-management techniques
- Provide post-rape interventions as described elsewhere in the text

G. Potential Outcomes

- May have no adverse outcomes if it is an isolated incident and with family, friends, and psychological support
- Sexually transmitted diseases
- Symptoms of PTSD, to include depression, anxiety, shame, sexual issues, isolation, despair, among numerous other psychological issues
- Excessive alcohol intake and its associated problems

"Instruction in sex is as important as instruction in food; yet not only are our adolescents not taught the physiology of sex, but never warned that the strongest sexual attractions may exist between persons so incompatible in tasks and capabilities that they could not endure living together for a week, much less a lifetime."

— George Bernard Shaw

2. Unintended Pregnancies in American Adolescents

A. Definition of Unintended Pregnancies. Pregnancies that occur in teenage girls who had unprotected sex during the fertile time in the girl's menstrual cycle. These pregnancies are often unplanned and are frequently unwanted by the girl and her partner.

B. Signs and Symptoms

- Unprotected sexual intercourse (absence of effective birth control use by the girl or her partner) during the girl's fertile sexual time
- The girl has stopped menstruating, has tender and enlarged breasts, slight weight gain (or weight loss if vomiting), abdominal girth gain, often nausea or vomiting, lightheadedness, and frequent urination
- Positive HCG serum/pregnancy test and ultrasound; bluish/purple colored vaginal walls, softening of the cervix, and enlargement of the uterus
- The adolescent may deny the presence of her pregnancy to herself, with frequent self-assertions that "*It cannot possibly be happening to me*"
- The girl may show signs of being worried, withdrawn,

moody, secretive, preoccupied, etc., or show emotions that are turbulent and actions that are out of character (allowing for the fact that she is also a teenager…)

C. Origins

- Minimal access exists for adolescents to obtain either reproductive health services, social support services, and low-cost contraceptives. These failures by society result in adolescents who are emotionally, physically, financially, and intellectually ill-prepared for the consequences of sexual intercourse[3]
- The youth of America today are being educated about sexuality by the mass media and their peers, rather than professionals; consequently, many of their vital questions go unanswered and misconceptions prevail
- With inappropriate sexual education, self-doubt, and mounting self, peer, and partner pressure to become sexually active, adolescents participate in sexual intercourse that is frequently not enjoyable and is awkward, painful, and unprotected
- Insufficient use of contraception methods, even though the numbers of youth who do use contraception has improved overall between 1991 and 2007 (their use of contraception went up from 46.2% to 61.5%)[4]

- The prevailing societal attitude in America today toward adolescent sexuality is to deny its very existence in the hope that if we ignore it and do not talk about it, perhaps it will just go away. Conversely, in many other nations (especially in most of Europe), a more open acceptance of teenage sexuality exists that is accompanied by very clear expectations and accountabilities by adolescents about their personal and community responsibilities when it comes to sex
- The stronger the mother/daughter relationship, the less chance the teen will engage in sexual intercourse and the greater chance for birth control use. Similarly, the more the mother appears to disapprove of the girl having sexual intercourse, the less likely it is that sexual intercourse will occur[5]
- Young children (under age 13) who engage in sexual intercourse have less likelihood to use contraception at first sexual intercourse, and often are a voluntary (willing), but unwanted (not at that time) participant at first sexual intercourse; there is an increased likelihood of adolescent birth; and these children experience an increased number of sexual partners during the adolescent years[6]

D. Background

- Every year, an estimated 750,000 adolescents become pregnant. The pregnancy rate for teenagers aged 15-19 fell 38% between 1990 and 2004; the lowest reported teen pregnancy rate since 1976. These pregnancies include live births, miscarriages, and abortions[4]
- Teen births declined from 1991 to 2005, but then rose 5% from 2005 to 2007[6]
- The decline in births to teens is mostly due to changes among African-American females' sexual activity; sexual activity among Caucasians and Hispanics remains unchanged
- Despite the decline in teen pregnancy in the United States, it remains one of the *highest* among industrialized nations[7]
- In a comparison of teenage sexual and reproductive behavior in five countries, the U.S., Canada, Great Britain, France, and Sweden, the U.S. teenage birthrate of 49 births per 1,000 women aged 15-19 (down about 20% from 1990), remains about twice as high as rates in Great Britain and Canada, and five times as high as in Sweden and France[8]
- Of high school students surveyed in 2011, 47.4% had sexual intercourse, 33.7% had sexual intercourse during

- the past three months, and of these, 39.8% did not use a condom the last time they had sex; 76.7% did not use birth control pills or Depo-Provera to prevent pregnancy the last time they had sex, and 15.3% had had sex with four or more people[9]
- Adolescents at a greater risk for early age pregnancy include those who live in a rural area, have parents on welfare, are African-American, and are from the South. Also, younger age, poor school performance, economic disadvantage, an older male partner, and single or teen parents also risk adolescent pregnancy[10]
- More than 400,000 teen girls aged 15-19 years in the U.S. gave birth in 2009[10]

E. Therapeutic Interventions

- Perform a Standard Sexual Assessment (Appendix C) and medical assessment, and obtain a sexual and medical history
- HCP to evaluate own sexuality and comfort with discussing sexuality with adolescents, and employ healthcare professionals who are also comfortable discussing sexuality with teens
- Develop an open attitude toward discussion of sexuality with teens, and actively engage them in meaningful

sexual conversation whenever the location and timing are appropriate
- Provide ante-natal care for the girl with careful observations for complications that may occur in adolescent girls. These include premature delivery, severe anemia, placenta praevia, and toxemia of pregnancy
- Provide prenatal care with additional monitoring for possible severe anemia, hypertension, nausea, and vomiting that leads to excessive weight loss
- Assess the girl for additional risk factors to health such as smoking, drug use, alcohol use, STDs, etc. Previous drug users often resume drug use within six months
- Encourage the girl to stay at school during pregnancy and post-delivery, and present the outcomes of not doing so
- Inform the girl, the baby's father, and her parents discreetly and non-judgmentally about future options for the baby, such as the mother raising her child alone, with the baby's father, with family support, adoption, or abortion

F. Supportive Interventions

- Review the Supportive Interventions Guide for Children (Appendix G)
- Develop/maintain education programs to prevent

adolescent pregnancies. These include abstinence only programs, education programs, abstinence and education programs, and peer counseling programs. However, research demonstrates that "abstinence only" programs are not effective in preventing early sexual intercourse, adolescent pregnancy, or STIs; however, combined with education programs, they reduce pregnancy risk factors

- Provide education to the girl regarding maternal and child health maintenance prior to delivery to include information about her dietary needs and those of her baby, the importance of exercise, and the use of contraceptives to prevent STDs
- Explain the hazards to her and her baby associated with smoking cigarettes and using drugs and alcohol
- Discuss breast-feeding and bottle-feeding equally, and include the negatives and positives of each method; allow the young woman to decide for herself
- Encourage attendance at organized childbirth classes
- Prepare the young woman for the birth of her baby. Explain in lay terms about the delivery room, the personnel, what to observe to determine when false labor and when actual labor begins, and what she can expect during the birth process. Describe her bodily changes that facilitate the baby's birth, the nursing and the medical procedures to expect, ways to lessen

contracture discomfort, and ways to enhance contracture effectiveness
- Monitor the young woman's contractions, administer analgesics as needed, and encourage and support the young woman in the advancement of the baby's journey. Monitor vital signs of the girl, and observe for signs of dehydration, toxemia, placenta praevia, excessive fatigue, and signs of fetal distress
- Support the young mother in her quest to remain in school
- Evaluate the relationship between the young woman and the baby's father, especially for the potential for partner violence

G. Potential Outcomes

- Girls who give birth at an early age often drop out of high school. The ramifications of this situation include insufficient education, inadequate work skills, limited problem-solving skills, inadequate social skills, future poverty, depression, and loneliness
- Adolescent fathers tend to have limited education, inadequate job skills, poorly paying jobs, and earn non-livable wages that do not adequately maintain their families

- Teen mothers are more likely to have unhealthy habits that place their infants at greater risk for inadequate growth, infection, or chemical dependence[10]
- Adolescent girls who are pregnant experience more complications associated with pregnancy and give birth to more low birth weight babies than older mothers
- Over 90% of girls who give birth choose to raise the baby, and 8% choose adoption
- Girls born to teen mothers are more likely to become teen mothers themselves. Boys born to teen mothers have a higher rate than other similar age boys of being jailed and arrested[11]
- Partner violence is the second leading cause of death during pregnancy for teen girls[12]

"Young people are moving away from feeling guilty about sleeping with somebody to feeling guilty if they are not sleeping with someone."

— Margaret Mead

3. Sexually Transmitted Infections (STIs) in American Adolescents

A. Definition. STIs are a wide range of infectious diseases that adolescents and others transmit through activities that are primarily sexual, either consensual or non-consensual, mostly sexual intercourse and the exchange of body fluids.

B. Signs and Symptoms

- Some STIs are asymptomatic but can be transmitted to a partner during sexual intercourse or body and body fluid contact
- Mayo Clinic[13] describes the signs and symptoms of frequently encountered STIs as including:

Chlamydia: painful urination, lower abdominal pain; vaginal discharge in women, penile discharge in men, painful sexual intercourse in women, and testicular pain in men

Gonorrhea: thick, lemon-colored, cloudy, or bloody discharge from the penis or vagina; pain on urination; abnormal menstrual bleeding; painful, swollen testicles; painful bowel movements; and anal itching
Trichomoniasis: transparent, white, greenish, yellowish vaginal discharge, a strong vaginal odor, vaginal itching, itching of the penis, penile discharge, painful intercourse, and painful urination

HIV: fever, headache, sore throat, swollen lymph glands, rash, and fatigue occur during first month or so. As the disease advances, and in ensuing months or more, symptoms such as diarrhea, swollen lymph nodes, weight loss, fever, cough, and shortness of breath occur. Later stage infection leads to persistent, unexplained fatigue, soaking night sweats, shaking chill, with elevated temperature, persistent swollen lymph nodes, chronic diarrhea, and unusual, opportunistic diseases

- According to the Family Planning Council[14], the signs and symptoms of other frequently encountered STIs include:

  - **Bacterial Vaginosis:** excessive and foul-smelling vaginal discharge
  - **Chancroid:** painful ulcers with reddened edges of the penis; painful, swollen lymph nodes of the groin; women may be asymptomatic
  - **Genital Warts:** single or multiple soft, fleshy skin lesions on the genitals and genital area, perineum, and anus
  - **Hepatitis:** yellowing of eyes and skin, abdominal pain, nausea and vomiting, fatigue, darkening urine or asymptomatic
  - **Genital Herpes 2:** burning pain while urinating, genital bumps and blisters, or asymptomatic

- **Human Papillomavirus:** Genital warts may appear, with genital skin changes, with genital itching, pain, or bleeding of the genital area
- **Pelvic Inflammatory Disease:** Women may have a white or yellow vaginal discharge, between period bleeding; heavier, painful periods; fevers, chills, nausea; and ectopic pregnancy

C. Origins

- Sometimes the origins of STIs are not fully understood; however, the origins of the majority of adverse STIs are caused by the presence and adverse effects of a known infectious organism in a man or woman

D. Background

- Sexually transmitted infections have been around for thousands of years and occur throughout the world. While a great deal of advanced knowledge about STIs is now available, they remain an onerous threat to society
- HPV infections account for the majority of newly acquired STIs, and about 90% of these will go away on their own in two years.[15] There is no treatment for the

- HPV itself, but there are for the diseases caused by HPV
- Risky sexual behaviors predispose adolescents to HIV infection and other STIs
- Earlier initiation of sexual intercourse is strongly associated with STIs of adolescents and young adults. The cervix of a younger adolescent is immature, which renders it and the girl susceptible and predisposed to infection during sexual intercourse
- Although America's youth represent 25% of the population, they account for nearly half of the new STIs; about 20 million a year[15]
- Adolescents who use drugs and alcohol are at greater risk for HIV, AIDS, and STIs because of unplanned and unprotected sex than non-drug users
- Males transmit STIs more effectively than women
- Each state has a list of required reportable diseases of great public health importance, some of which are STIs, and state personnel monitor and report on their identified cases of STIs[16]

E. Therapeutic Interventions

- Perform a Standard Sexual Assessment (Appendix C) and medical assessment, and obtain a sexual and medical history

- Be aware of the five major strategies (guidelines) by CDC for STD/HIV prevention and ensure that they are used to guide interventions implemented.[17(p2)] These include: a.) education and counseling of persons at risk on ways to avoid STDs through changes in sexual behaviors and use of recommended prevention services; b.) identification of asymptomatic infected persons and of symptomatic persons unlikely to seek diagnostic and treatment services; c.) effective diagnosis, treatment, and counseling of infected persons; evaluation, treatment, and counseling of sex partners for persons who are infected with an STD; and pre-exposure vaccination of persons at risk for vaccine-preventable STDs
- Obtain a history from the adolescent (especially history of contributing factors), and perform all required diagnostic tests on the adolescent before beginning any therapy
- Ensure tests for commonly occurring STIs (e.g., chlamydia) are done before those that occur less frequently (e.g., syphilis); where there is one STI there are almost invariably more
- Perform visual inspection of vulva, penis, perineum, anus, and observe for discharge, odor, scrotum, urethra, bleeding, irritation, warts, ulcerative lesions, and signs of trauma
- Obtain swabs from the pharynx and anus of the boy or

girl, vagina of the girl and urethra in the boy, and test for gonorrhea and trachomatis; take a culture and test for frequently occurring STIs
- Four STIs are relatively easily treated and cured if diagnosed early: chlamydia, gonorrhea, syphilis, and trichomoniasis
- Refer to an expert in HIV and AIDs care if positive results obtained, and determine what therapies are needed. Refer to CDC guidelines for treatment of STIs/HIV (2010)[18] and order appropriately
- Promote increased access to sexual and reproductive healthcare services for adolescents
- Participate in changing social attitudes toward increased acceptance of adolescent sexuality together with education about sexual responsibility, personal commitment, and accountability
- Educate adolescents, their parents, and the community about transmission and prevention of sexual infections

F. Supportive Interventions

- Review the Supportive Interventions Guide for Adults (Appendix H)
- Collaborate with the physician or FNP to determine the priority of the STI and the need to involve the adolescent's parents

- Obtain or assist the MD/FNP with specimen collection and specimen identification
- Monitor adolescent that all vital signs are within normal limits
- Administer prescribed antibiotics, anti-virals, vaccines, etc.
- If receive confirmation that STI test is positive, notify the state registry of the incidence with associated details
- Assure the adolescent of absolute confidentiality and privacy
- Develop and implement safety measures for the adolescent if forced sex determined
- Determine the adolescent's level of understanding of the offending STI and teach accordingly
- Teach the adolescent about medications, treatments, appointments, vaccinations, blood levels, and overall management of the infection involved
- Teach about efficacy of contraception in STI prevention and answer all questions in age-appropriate language
- If father, mother, or sibling is the adult who sexually abused the adolescent, notify state and child welfare authorities and arrange for alternate placement
- Promote increased access to sexual and reproductive healthcare services for adolescents to participate in changing social attitudes toward increased acceptance

of adolescent sexuality together with education about sexual responsibility, personal commitment, and accountability
- Educate adolescents, their parents, and the community about transmission and prevention of sexual infections

G. Potential Outcomes

If the treatment protocol is continued and completed, the outcome for the adolescent is usually excellent. Issues arise when the risky behavior of the adolescent continues, as untreated or incompletely treated STIs may progress to ongoing multiple infections, sterility, ectopic pregnancy, pelvic inflammatory disease in girls, malignancy, and other life-threatening diseases.

"As the world confronts the challenges of globalization, the entertainment industry, a web saturated with explicit sexual content, is increasingly making it difficult for young people to make informed decisions about sex."

— Oche Otorkpa

4. Rape in American Adolescents

4a. Definition of Rape. "Rape is a criminal offense defined in most states as forcible sexual relations, especially sexual intercourse, with a person against that person's will."[18(p1)] However, some states carefully define the type of contact that constitutes rape. For example, Hawaii's state law defines sexual penetration as "vaginal intercourse, anal intercourse, fellatio, cunnilingus, analingus, deviate sexual intercourse, or any part of a person's body or of any object into the genital or anal opening of another person's body... however slight."[18(p3)]

4b. Definition of Acquaintance Rape (to include Date Rape). "Acquaintance assault involves coercive activities that occur against a person's will by means of force, violence, duress, or fear of bodily injury. These sexual activities are imposed upon them by someone they know as a friend, date, acquaintance, etc."[19] In acquaintance rape, the victim usually knows her assailant fairly, moderately, or very well. In college, the victim knows 9 in 10 offenders. Most often a boyfriend, ex-boyfriend, classmate, friend, acquaintance, or co-worker sexually assaults the woman.[19 (p1,para1)]

189

Acquaintance rape includes military rape, statutory rape, spousal or partner rape, and gang rape; names given that reflect the victim's relationship with the offender or the circumstances in which the rape occurred. Date rape usually occurs at the end of a first date, so the assailant is not very well-known to the adolescent.[19]

4c. Definition of Stranger Rape. Rape that is executed by an assailant who is usually not known by the victim and with whom no prior relationship exists; he mostly attacks his victim in a dark, isolated place with a planned exit route and minimal chance of being caught. Violence toward the victim is often involved.[19]

B₁. Signs and Symptoms of Acquaintance Rape

- The young woman may or may not show visible signs of distress; she may be disheveled, have signs of a struggle and resistance, and signs of injury, or her appearance and demeanor may not indicate any of these signs
- She is often in a state of disbelief and denial that her acquaintance or friend has done this to her; perceived as a violation of trust as well as physical assault

- She may later demonstrate a few or more signs/symptoms to include: embarrassment, guilt, irritability, and moodiness; self-blame rather than blame assailant for what happened; anxiety, helplessness, low self-esteem, anger, and humiliation

B₂. Signs and Symptoms of Stranger Rape

- After the rape, the girl may or may not tell her parents or her family about the rape; however, she often tells her closest friends, but rarely notifies the authorities
- The girl is in a state of agitation, often with obvious signs of emotional and physical distress, or remains silent, withdrawn, and non-communicative

C. Origins

- Rape has been typified by researchers according to characteristics of the rapist, the victim, and/or the situation. Groth[20] (1979) first described three types of rapists based on the rapist's goals and characteristics—anger rapist, power rapist, and sadistic rapist

  - **Anger Rapists** seek to disperse anger and hostility

that has built up over time, to debase victims through degrading and humiliating acts, and will use profane language and considerable physical force to cause serious harm to their victims. The anger rapist rapes spontaneously, and rape is usually precipitated by a distressing life event for the rapist
- **Power Rapists** are motivated by power, and need to control and possess their victims more than cause them physical bodily harm. They feel inadequate and insecure in their masculinity and manhood, so they seek to conquer and possess women in an effort to show their manhood does exist. They have the belief that the victim may resist, but she actually enjoys the rape. Planning and thought goes into this type of rape[20]
- **Sadistic Rapists** are the most dangerous of all rapists. They experience sexual pleasure from sadistic acts against their victim, and they are abusive. During the act of rape, they often mutilate or even kill their victims. These rapes are well-planned, and stalking of the victim may be involved[20]
- Rapes are also classified according to the characteristics of the victim and any relationship that the victim may or may not have with the victim; these are divided into two groups, acquaintance rapist or stranger rapist

High Risk Sexual Behaviors

- **Acquaintance Rapists** have some prior relationship with the victim. The rape names include date rape, marital rape, military rape, gang rape, prison rape, statutory rape, and corrective rape. It has been suggested that acquaintance rape is about sexual attraction, sexual passion, sexual gratification, and the inability of the perpetrator to stop the act; this is not supported by research. Rape is an act of control, aggression, domination, and violence, with some element of sexuality[20]
- **Stranger Rapists** have no relationship whatsoever with their victims, and the victim does not know the assailant. The assault is often planned, with victim selection, following the potential victim, and escape route planning. Violence toward the victim is involved[20]

D. **Background**

- Rape is a serious crime that is underreported by girls and women for many reasons, including: fear of disbelief by police, perpetration of the act by a friend or relative, the perception that girls and women enjoy being raped, fear of hospital examinations, fear of the legal system, fear of reprisal by the assailant, and self-blame and shame

- According to many states' laws, there are four degrees of sexual assault (rape), the criteria for which are usually described in detail
- An average of 237,868 Americans above the age of 12 years are raped each year.[19] One in 33 of these are men
- 60% of rapes are never reported to the police, and 97% of rapists never spend any time in jail for the assault
- It is estimated that almost 25% of college women have been victims of rape or attempted rape since the age of 14.[21] "Women ages 16 to 24 experience rape at four times higher than the assault rate on all women, making the college years the most vulnerable for women."[22]
- Very little data is available on the rape of individuals within the LGBTQ communities. Not only is theirs a community that remains stigmatized but also one that is ignored, as demonstrated by the lack of support, lack of resources, and lack of LGBTQ rape-research.
- Most rapes are executed on girls and women by men; women on women rapes are infrequent; however, males are also victims of rapists, primarily by males. Women on men sexual assault is usually in the form of unwanted sexual touching, rubbing up against, hugging, kissing, etc. However, few men report sexual incidences to the authorities
- "Despite the violation and reality of physical and

emotional trauma, victims of acquaintance assault often do not identify their experience as sexual assault. Instead of focusing on the violation of the sexual assault, victims of acquaintance rape often blame themselves for the assault"[21(p1)]
- Many men and women still view acquaintance rape as an activity that the woman enjoys, and willingly participates in, even though there may be extreme violence involved
- Drugs such as Rohypnol (*roofies*) and gamma hydroxybutyrate (*GHB*), and alcohol make rape much easier for the potential rapist. When ingested, these result in a reduction of the teen's inhibitions, clear-thinking, and reduce decision-making skills; produce a loss of consciousness and amnesia; and often play a role in the attempt and completion of chemically-related rapes
- A current or former relationship between two individuals, either sexual or non-sexual, does *not* constitute an agreement for them to have sexual intercourse. Neither does the wearing of provocative clothing, flirtatious behavior, or being alone with another person

E. Therapeutic Interventions

- Perform a Standard Sexual Assessment (Appendix C) and medical assessment, and obtain a sexual and medical history
- Convene rape crisis team (if available); if not, the physician and nurse with experience in rape crisis interventions are assigned, as well as a psychologist
- Provide support and understanding, and avoid any demonstration of personal feelings or judgment. Deliver questions quietly and avoid any that lead or confuse
- Obtain sexual, medical, family, and social assessments
- Perform a head-to-toe physical assessment, to include an anal-genital exam for bruising, bleeding, trauma, lacerations, and anal dilatation, among others
- Obtain cultures of throat, blood, or body lesions for presence of STIs; obtain photographs; and trace forensic evidence collection if possible
- Assess for signs of pregnancy
- Assess for presence of Rohypnol and hydroxybutyrate as well as other illicit drugs
- Determine what type of psychological issues are present
- Prescribe analgesics, sedatives, if needed
- Determine whether there is a need for psychological or psychiatric interventions, and if needed, determine

the type of supportive therapy that might benefit the young woman

F[1]. Supportive Interventions (Preventative)

- Review the Supportive Interventions Guide for Adults (Appendix H)
- Encourage healthcare facility administrators to budget for and create an additional position for a family nurse practitioner (FNP), a rape crisis counselor, a forensic nurse examiner (FNE), or a sexual assault nurse examiner (SANE) to ensure that the victim is examined and cared for by experienced personnel.
- Implement, teach, and reinforce rape prevention programs in healthcare facilities, high schools, middle schools, and colleges that provide the adolescents, young adults, and their parents with the rape-avoidance tools they need. These programs, directed specifically to the youth in the audience, should include topics such as:
  - The statistics and circumstances of types of acquaintance rape and stranger rape
  - Methods by which young people can maintain themselves in positions of safety
  - Provide sexual education programs that dispel the myths and promote the truths associated with rape

information
- Encourage adolescents to listen to their gut feelings of fear and discomfort when any situation does not feel right, and remove self from the vicinity
- Promote non-use of alcohol and drugs by teens, and minimal use of alcohol by young women and young men, especially in a college environment
- Teach avoidance of places where there is no access to an exit, another person, and/or means of assistance; always carry a cell-phone or have access to a phone, tell friends or family of destination and plans, and share name with others of person going to meet
- Advise to attend schools or colleges with anti-sexual violence policies and programs in place that emphasize rape prevention and that also publish the effectiveness of their programs
- Provide adolescents with the names of sexual assault crisis centers and hotlines to call in a time of crisis
- If rape occurs, advise the victim to go immediately to the closest hospital, call the local rape hotline, or go to a rape crisis center. Caution not to change clothes or shower to facilitate evidence collection

F². Post-Rape Supportive Interventions

- Review the Supportive Interventions Guide for Children (Appendix G) and Adults (Appendix H)
- If experience and knowledge are insufficient, request a different assignment and gain necessary education and experience in preparation for the next assignment
- Obtain a sexual history without use of leading questions or prompting the young woman
- Ensure that the young woman is comfortable, without pain, warm, vital signs stable, and afebrile
- Treat any lacerations or abrasions and observe for other bodily trauma
- Administer fluids orally and/or intravenously
- Work closely with the other HCPs in all aspects of the post-rape workup process to include specimen collection, blood collection, photographs, vaginal examination
- Notify next of kin, and obtain their contact information
- Notify authorities of sexual assault

G. Potential Outcomes

- Some post-rape individuals see themselves as survivors rather than victims and are able to function as well if

not better than prior to rape without any untoward outcomes
- Ongoing and persistent fear for her personal safety as the victim is forced on a daily basis to see the assailant at school, in college, and in the community
- Acquaintance rape victims suffer the same psychological harms as stranger rape victims: shock, humiliation, anxiety, depression, substance abuse, suicidal ideation, loss of self-esteem, social isolation[22]
- PTSD (with flashbacks and adverse memories) is 6 times more likely and alcohol abuse 13 times more likely in young women post-rape[22]
- Guilt, shame, and self-blame may occur, accompanied by self-harm and self-isolation, as well as anger toward self and others
- Physical conditions such as urinary tract infections and STIs to include gonorrhea, genital warts, and chlamydia often occur
- Physical injuries such as vaginal and anal tears that may result in local infection, pelvic infection, vaginitis, vulvodynia, and dyspareunia
- Frequently young women are the unfortunate recipients of *victim blame* from the community school officials, healthcare personnel, and law enforcement

SECTION 4

SEXUAL ISSUES THAT MAY RESULT FROM SEXUAL ORIENTATION, GENDER IDENTITY DYSPHORIA, AND/OR SEX DEVELOPMENTAL VARIANCES

CHAPTER 6

PROBLEMS THAT ADULTS AND ADOLESCENTS WHO ARE GAY, LESBIAN, OR BISEXUAL EXPERIENCE AS A RESULT OF THEIR SEXUAL ORIENTATION

"Another lesson for me, twenty years ago, was equally clear: there is no justification ever, for the degrading, the debasing or the exploitation of other human beings-on whatever basis: nationality, race, ethnicity, religion, gender, sexual orientation, disability, age or caste."

— Zeid Ra'ad Al Hussein (U.N.)

According to the American Psychological Association,[1(p1)] "Sexual orientation refers to the sex of those to whom one is sexually and romantically attracted." Sexual orientation also refers to a person's sense of identity based on those attractions, related behaviors, and membership in a community of others who share these attractions. Research over several decades has demonstrated that sexual orientation ranges along a continuum, from exclusive attraction to the other sex to exclusive attraction to the same sex. However, sexual orientation is usually discussed in terms of three categories: a) heterosexual (having emotional, romantic, or sexual attractions to members of the other sex), b) gay/lesbian (having emotional, romantic, or sexual attractions to members of one's own sex), and c) bisexual (having emotional, romantic, or sexual attractions to both men and women).

Note: Information on persons of transgender follows later in the gender identity section.

A. Definitions.

A_1. A gay person is a boy or man, who is sexually and affectionately attracted to males. He may/may not be sexually active with other males

A_2. A lesbian is a girl or woman, who is sexually and affectionately attracted to other females. She may or may not be sexually active with other females

A_3. A bisexual person is a man or a woman who is sexually and affectionately attracted to both men and women

B_1 Signs and Symptoms Specific to Gay Youth, Adult Gay

Males, and Bisexual Males

- Higher rates of major depression, generalized anxiety, and substance abuse or dependence occurs in lesbian and gay youth and gay men, with higher rates of suicidal thoughts among gay youth than heterosexual youth, but approximately the same rates for actual suicide attempts. Higher rates of use of mental health services are seen among gay men and lesbians[2]
- Isolation, alienation, and withdrawal (self or externally imposed)
- Interpersonal, work, and school-related problems
- Family conflict between adolescents and parents, siblings, or adults with the partner, parents, siblings, and others
- Eating disorders and nutritional deficiencies occur
- High rates of malignancies exist, malignancies that include "lung and stomach, as well as anal/rectal cancer, Kaposi's sarcoma, and cancer of the breast, endometrial, and ovarian cancer. Also, sexually transmitted diseases are seen such as herpes, hepatitis B, syphilis, human papilloma virus, chlamydia, gonorrhea and HIV and AIDS"[3(p39)]
- Prostitution by young males related to being a runaway, homeless, and without money or support systems

- Reduced or absent access to healthcare services, to include sex-related education, health assessment, and screening; therapy, counseling, clinics, follow-up, and prevention

B₂. Causes of Signs and Symptoms Specific to Gay Youth, Adult Gay Males, and Bisexual Males

- Adult gay males, adolescent gay males, and bisexual people experience many adverse conditions because of their sexual orientation which account for a number of signs and symptoms they present. These include: mild to severe homophobia (fear, hatred, and an irrational fear of all that is GLB related) or biphobia
- Prejudice and discrimination exist in employment, housing, and stereotyping, among others; verbal and physical harassment, individual or gang violence, bullied at school, and intentionally *outed* without the person's permission; absence of partner acknowledgment or recognition, and denial of decision-making participation
- Race, ethnicity, religion, disability, economic status, and level of education may exacerbate the abuse inflicted and adverse effects experienced
- Internalization of negative stereotyping occurs in some persons who are gay or lesbian as they unconsciously

internalize much of the negative stereotyping that they repeatedly hear about gays or lesbians; they come to believe that it is true, and self-dislike or even self-hatred may follow
- High-risk activities such as excessive smoking related to lung cancer, unprotected sex, excessive alcohol, and use of drugs that might result in sexually transmitted infections, alcoholism, liver damage, and even death
- Perceived and actual homophobia and biphobia of healthcare professionals, societal stigma, and stereotyping that leads to avoidance of healthcare personnel and environment

B₃. Signs and Symptoms Specific to Adolescent and Adult Lesbians and Bisexual Women

Most lesbians and bisexual women lead healthy lives. However, some health problems are more common among lesbian and bisexual women than among heterosexual women. These include heart disease, cancer, depression, smoking, alcohol and drug use, sexually transmitted diseases (bacterial vaginosis, genital herpes, human papilloma virus, pubic lice, trichomoniasis; gonorrhea, hepatitis B, and HIV/AIDS are less likely), polycystic ovary syndrome, and domestic violence[4]

B₄. Causes of Signs and Symptoms Specific to Adolescent and Adult Lesbians and Bisexual Women

- Lesbian and bisexual women have a higher rate of obesity, smoking, and stress than heterosexual women, all of which contribute to heart disease; lesbians and bisexual women are less likely to get Pap tests; the viruses that cause most cervical cancer can be sexually transmitted woman to woman.[4] Bisexual and lesbian women are less likely to have medical insurance. Depression may be due to social stigma, rejection by family members, abuse and violence, unfair treatment by the legal system, stress from hiding their sexual orientation, and lack of health insurance
- The group most likely to smoke are bisexual women, while lesbians are more likely to smoke than heterosexual women due to stress, low self-esteem, anxiety due to hiding sexual orientation, and tobacco ads aimed at gays and lesbians
- Marazzo et al.[4] found that women with only female partners in the previous two months had 3.4 partners in the past year, and women with male and female partners had 16.5 partners in the past year. Women who report sex with both men and women are likely to be at highest risk for STIs

Gay, Lesbian or Bisexual Problems

- Lesbian and bisexual women may have male partners who are at higher risk for HIV and STIs than the partners of women who have sex with men only[3]
- Alcohol drinking has decreased among lesbians; however, it and drug use continue to be elevated. This reduction may be due to a small decrease in the social stigma and the changing norm among some lesbian groups[4]
- It is suggested that lesbians may have a higher rate of polycystic ovarian disease than heterosexual women due to excess androgen
- Domestic violence occurs in lesbian relationships as well as in heterosexual relationships; however, the rate may be higher because lesbians tend to remain silent through fear of reprisal, loss of children, and fear of discrimination

C. Origins

- No one knows what causes heterosexuality, homosexuality, or bisexuality. Homosexuality was once thought to be a result of troubled family dynamics or faulty psychological development, but this theory was later felt to be based upon assumptions made from misinformation and prejudice

- Several factors have been identified to indicate that a number of biological influences may be involved in the origins of sexual orientation, to include genetics, prenatal hormones, and brain structure, and social, developmental, and environmental influences are also believed to be involved. No one factor has been identified as the main determinant of sexual orientation
- "Despite almost a century of psychoanalytic speculation, there is no evidence to support the suggestion that the nature of parenting or early childhood experiences play any role in the formation of a person's heterosexual or homosexual orientation. It seems that sexual orientation is biological in nature, determined by a complex interplay of genetic factors and early uterine environment. Sexual orientation is, therefore, not a choice, though sexual behavior is"[5(p6)]

D. Background

- The term *sexual orientation* is neither a clinical nor a legal term; there is no term that is accepted by psychologists to describe clearly and adequately sexual orientation
- Lesbian, gay, and bisexual sexual orientations are not

Gay, Lesbian or Bisexual Problems

disorders; their relationships are a normal form of human experience and human bonding[6(p3)]
- Legal changes have been made in an effort to reduce the adverse perceptions and actions against people who are gay, lesbian, or bisexual; however, in direct interactions, discrimination toward lesbian, gay, and bisexual people persists
- Bisexual individuals not only experience discrimination from heterosexual people, but they also are discriminated against by some lesbians and gay men. They also experience discrimination by healthcare professionals and frequently fear reprisals and inadequate care
- Health issues of people who are LGB are treated as inconsequential because they only affect a few people compared to the greater number of heterosexual patients
- Some healthcare professionals provide inadequate and cursory care to people who are LGB, give negative responses, provide rushed and unprofessional examinations and procedures, and interact in an off-hand, rude manner
- Myths and stereotypes abound about people who are gay, lesbian, or bisexual, including:
    - *AIDS is a gay disease.* Not true: even though many

gay men have been infected. It is a viral disease, relatively easy to transmit, that infects all kinds of people regardless of their gender, biological sex, or sexual orientation
- *Since Alfred Kinsey's research in 1948 and 1954, the prevalence of people of a gay or lesbian (more or less exclusively homosexual) sexual orientation has been accepted as being about 10% of males and 2.6% of women.* However, according to the Kinsey Institute, in a study that involved 3,432 men and women, Laumann et al. indicate that the frequency of *some level of homosexuality* is 2.8% for males, and 1.4% for women[7(p3)]
- *The relationships of lesbians and gay men are dysfunctional and unhappy.* Studies have found that same-sex and heterosexual couples are equivalent to each other on measures of relationship satisfaction and commitment[6(p4)]
- *Lesbians and gay men flit from one sexual encounter to another, are promiscuous, and do not want a committed relationship.* Research demonstrates that many lesbians and gay men want and have committed relationships; 40-60% of gay men and 45-80% of lesbians are currently involved in a romantic relationship, and 1 in 9

couples who are living together have partners of the same sex.[6(p4)] They are no more or no less promiscuous than heterosexuals
- *Being gay, lesbian, or bisexual is a mental condition.* It is not, although mental problems may arise as a result of adverse societal treatment. In 1973, The American Psychiatric Association removed homosexuality from its list of mental disorders, and identified homosexuality to be as healthy as heterosexuality
- *If a lesbian couple adopts or a lesbian woman gives birth to a baby, or a gay couple adopts a child and they rear that child, that child will grow up to be lesbian or gay and have gender role and identification problems.* Research shows that sexual identities develop the same way among children of lesbian parents as they do among heterosexual parents
- *Nature supersedes nurture or nurture supersedes nature in the origin of sexual orientation.* Most likely sexual orientation is a combination of both biological and environmental influences
- *All gay people are pedophiles.* This myth is not supported by research; homosexual males are no more likely to molest children than are heterosexual

males. According to Herek[8], in a 1970s national survey, more than 70% of respondents agreed with the assertion that "homosexuals are dangerous as teachers because they try to get sexually involved with children, or that homosexuals attempt to play sexually with children if they cannot get an older partner."[8(Blog,p1,paras5,6)] By contrast, in the 1999 national poll, the belief that the gayest men are likely to molest or abuse children was endorsed by only 19% of men, and 10% of heterosexual women. Similarly, Jenny et al.[9] did not find a connection between child molesters and homosexuality. In their review of 352 medical records of children who had been molested, the molester was a gay or lesbian adult in fewer than 1% of cases in which an adult molester could be identified—only 2 out of 269 cases

- *Lesbians have low self-esteem.* This myth is also not supported by research. Lesbians reported equally strong levels of mental health as their heterosexual sisters and higher self-esteem[2]

E. Therapeutic Interventions

- Perform a standard new patient medical workup

(include routine blood work as indicated); obtain a sexual health and sexual health history from self-identified lesbian, gay, or bisexual patients. Include the use of sexual orientation tools such as *The Klein Sexual Orientation Grid*,[10] and the seven point *Kinsey Sexual Orientation Scale*,[11] among others

- Be sensitive to the cultural differences of patients and learn about those differences; acknowledge personal biases, use of stereotyping; accept own sexuality and personal sexual issues
- Be sensitive to any provider-based barriers to LGB healthcare within the practice and manage them appropriately
- Become educated about homosexuality and bisexuality and the associated health and life problems patients may have to face
- Identify and document staff deficiencies in LGB-specific knowledge needs, and educate staff to meet those needs through sensitivity training, empathy training, and LGB language awareness
- Develop office literature that uses LGB-sensitive language and provides information about topics such as: patient rights, intake pre-procedures/procedures, care procedures, confidentiality, privacy, healthcare follow-up, informed consent, partner visitation and

participation, health education, and associated health problems
- Assure patients of confidentiality and privacy, as well as a reduction in the number of tests and examinations that involve disrobing and intense observation and scrutiny by others
- Encourage employees to challenge the witnessed homophobia of others, evaluate their levels of heterosexism and homophobia, and promote an open attitude toward sexual diversity
- Perform necessary tests according to the findings of the verbal history, sexual orientation tools, physical assessment and identified areas of concern, and treat all problems that warrant attention; problems such as those identified in previous sections
- Initiate support services such as dietary support, social services, family support services, financial services, and child protective services as needed; refer patient to specialized healthcare professionals such as a psychologist, oncologist, HIV/AIDS specialist, public health services, substance abuse counselor, and STI specialist; prescribe medications for the identified problems, as well as vaccines for Hepatitis A and B for all gay and bisexual men examined
- Discourage Reparative or Conversion Therapy

(therapy to change the sexual orientation of a person who is gay, lesbian, or bisexual to a heterosexual orientation) as it *not* a medical option; it is neither safe nor effective and is harmful to the individual

F. Supportive Interventions

- Review the Supportive Interventions Guide for Adults (Appendix H)
- HCP managers must develop and implement non-discrimination policies for healthcare professionals when they care for patients who are in a sexual minority; monitor, demand compliance, and manage non-compliance equitably, rapidly, and firmly
- Discourage the use of heterosexism and heteronormism (the assumption that society is heterosexual and superior to other sexual orientations) within the healthcare environment
  Discuss with LGB adolescents about the feelings, challenges, and successes of adolescent sexuality
- Educate LGB adolescents regarding risky sexual, drug, and alcohol-related behaviors
- Treat all LGB youth as ordinary adolescents
- Many gays and lesbians (not usually bisexuals) choose to *come out* while many others choose to keep their

sexual orientation private. Avoid attempts to persuade or cajole the gay or lesbian person; the coming out process is a very personal decision and requires much thought
- Inform gay and lesbian patients that research shows that the *coming out* process may be daunting (especially for adolescents), yet when initiated, often promotes increased self-confidence, higher self-esteem, and personal satisfaction and fulfillment
- If person has decided to come out, support and assist adolescents and adults during the *coming out* process, a life-changing process that involves two steps. First, coming out to oneself, and second, coming out to one's family, friends, and even strangers that one's sexual orientation is not heterosexual
- There is no set time or age for coming out to occur, but the age appears to be getting younger, sometimes before a person is mentally and socially equipped to overcome some of the difficulties. Entering college and leaving parental oversight is often the first time one will acknowledge and act according to sexual orientation
- Educate colleagues, other healthcare professionals and non-professionals, and members of the public about the facts associated with homosexuality and bisexuality

Gay, Lesbian or Bisexual Problems

- Dispel the myths that all gay men are pedophiles, mentally ill, lack commitment to a monogamous, stable sexual relationship, are always *getting it on* sexually, only interested in hanging out in bars and picking up young men, or being picked up by older men, are bad parents, among others
- Dispel the myths that lesbians lack commitment to a monogamous, stable sexual relationship
- Assist in all procedures where indicated

G. Potential Outcomes

- It is difficult to determine what the outcomes will be for persons who are gay, lesbian, or bisexual because discrimination, with its adverse impact potential, continues to be a serious issue. However, current trends in activities and poll findings indicate that increased approval of LGBT persons is now apparent
- A USA Today/Gallup poll[13] demonstrates that Americans overall and LGBT adults are positive when asked how challenging it is for gay or lesbian adults to live in their community. A majority in each group say *it is not too difficult* or *not at all difficult* to live as openly gay. However, about 40% of each group believe it is difficult to do so where they live

- Sixty-three percent of Americans describe discrimination against gays and lesbians as a serious or somewhat serious problem in the U.S., while 88% of Americans who are LGBT see discrimination as a serious problem[13]
- "The poll finds 91% of adults saying people in their community have become more accepting of gays and lesbians in recent years;"[13] Gallup trends on gay and lesbian rights indicate a growing acceptance and tolerance in recent decades, especially among younger adults. Gallup also found that a majority of Americans now favor same-sex marriage, whereas in 2011, a majority opposed same-sex marriage
- However, Gallup[13] also finds that a slim majority, 51%, say the public will eventually agree on gay rights issues in the future; but nearly as many, 45%, believe these issues will always divide Americans. However, LGBT adults are more optimistic and believe that 77% will agree in the future

Note: As of October 6, 2014, 50% of states have legal same-sex marriage, and 25 states still have same-sex bans.[13]

CHAPTER 7

SEXUAL AND SOCIAL PROBLEMS THAT ADULTS AND ADOLESCENTS WITH GENDER DYSPHORIA ENCOUNTER

"As men and women of conscience, we reject discrimination in general, and in particular based on sexual orientation and gender identity. Where there is tension between cultural attitudes and human rights, human rights carry the day."

— Ban Ki-moon (U.N.)

Transgender is a term inclusive of a range of transgender, transsexual, and gender-variant identities of people who no longer express or identity their gender with their natal (birth) sex. Transgender people include transgender women (natal males with a feminine gender identity), sometimes referred to as male-to-females, or MTFs; transgender men (natal females with a masculine gender identity), sometimes referred to as female-to-males, or FTMs: and others who self-identify using one or some of the 100 known terms, including many that extend beyond the traditional gender binary choices.[1]

Note: The majority of information that follows is about the adult perspective associated with gender dysphoria as many of the same aspects of gender dysphoria (GD) are shared by both adolescents and adults. Where there are differences for adolescents, these are differentiated, either by further information or bold font.

A. **Definition.** DSM-5 (2013) refers to GD (previously gender identity disorder), as a marked incongruence between one's experienced or expressed gender and assigned agenda, of at least six months duration, as manifested by two or more of the following indicators:[2]

   a. a marked incongruence between one's experienced and expressed gender and secondary sex characteristics, or **in young adolescents, their anticipated secondary sex characteristics**
   b. a strong desire to be rid of one's primary and secondary sex characteristics because of a marked incongruence with one's experienced or expressed gender (**or, in young adolescents, a desire to prevent the development of the anticipated secondary sex characteristics**)
   c. a strong desire for the primary and secondary sex

characteristics of the other gender
d. a strong desire to be of and treated as the other gender (or some alternative gender, different from one's assigned gender)
e. a strong conviction that one has the typical feelings and reactions of the other gender (or some alternative gender different from the assigned gender)

B. Signs and Symptoms

- Presence of two or more of the above indicators
- Adults display symptoms of gender dysphoria that are both similar and different from those of children. They desire to live as a person in the opposite sex, be free of their own genitals, dress and behave as a person in the opposite sex; they suffer feelings of anxiety, isolation, loneliness, depression, distress, and sometimes suicidal thoughts as a result of those desires
- May demonstrate or complain of having been harassed, discriminated against, and being the recipient of assault
- The amount of personal distress experienced varies from person to person, from mild to severe; not all persons of transgender have distress. However, most persons of transgender will experience some emotional upheaval associated with gender dysphoria at one time

or another
- Transphobia may be internalized, and with it comes shame, guilt, blame, and self-hating as well as hatred of other transgender persons
- Gender dysphoric adolescents are a *heterogenous group* who may ask for sex reassignment but with ambivalence; have a strong desire for sex reassignment during the intake phase, but change their minds later; have no sex reassignment request, but are confused about their gender feelings; have gender concerns secondary to a co-existing condition"[3]
- Elevated levels of high-risk behaviors, e.g., prostitution (often as a result of poverty), intravenous drug use, and unprotected receptive anal or vaginal sex have been reported among transgender people, especially transgender women. "The HIV/AIDs epidemic has had a devastating impact on transgender people."[4(p3)] "HIV infection is highest among transgender women of color; African-American transgender women ranging from 41 to 63 percent and Latina transgender women from 14 to 50 percent"
- Gender dysphoric adolescents also have a high rate of HIV, although the actual percentage is difficult to determine as many transgender youths are homeless, transient, and not readily available for clinical studies

C. Origins

- The exact cause or origin of gender dysphoria has not been identified, but many theories have been proposed and the search goes on. These include a) internal influences within the fetus very early in utero (nature, biology), b) external influences that occur in the child after birth (nurture, environment), and/or c) internal biological influences that interact with external environmental influences
- Theories suggested include a *disconnect* between the brain sex differentiation and genital sex differentiation; a chromosomal or hormonal imbalance in the fetus during development; defects in human bonding, socialization, and child rearing; difference in brain volumes between individuals with GD and standard males; maternal stress hormones or medications; and autogynephilic males who desire to interact with themselves in a female body

D. Background

- The frequency of transgenderism is rare; however, some consider it to occur more frequently and estimate it to be 2-5% of the population[5]

- Lack of healthcare insurance, unemployment or underemployment, loss of viable income, and lack of support are just some of the challenges faced by persons of transgender
- The adverse impact of a stigma, discrimination, isolation, persecution, marginalization, violence, etc., often results in psychiatric illness
- Over the last two decades, the social climate overall toward adolescents and adults with GD may have improved slightly in America (more so in Europe) as people become more aware of the above. However, violence in the form of physical and sexual assault against persons of transgender in the U.S. continues to be high
- Persons of transgender with or without gender dysphoria are underserved by the healthcare community membership for reasons above, as well as a lack of preparation and education, insensitivity, and understanding of people of transgender by healthcare professionals, both during their education and their work environment
- Avoidance of healthcare professionals and facilities by people of transgender results in limited access to acute or preventative healthcare services, social services, and numerous other support services

- Family members may be unreceptive to the person of transgender, especially fathers toward their son's transgender behavior; mothers are usually more receptive and understanding
- Many persons with GD may not seek hormone transition therapy or surgery; instead, they try to integrate and celebrate their masculine and feminine selves through an androgynous or bi-gendered person

E. Therapeutic Interventions

- Perform a Standard Sexual Assessment (Appendix C) and medical assessment, and obtain psychosocial, psychosexual, and medical histories
- Perform physical assessment that centers on the organs of the patient rather than the perceived organs of the patient; it is the existing organs, not the perceived organs, that may be or may become diseased
- Blood screening performed depends on the patient's transition status and the diseases that frequently occur during and after transition. For example, male to female (MTF) persons have their increased risk for coronary artery disease due to estrogen and the presence of hypertension, diabetes, obesity, venous thrombosis and embolism, and smoking

- Normal values for individuals undergoing gender transition have not been established[6]
- Inform lab personnel that appearance may not match the sex identified on the lab form, and may or may not be compared to established blood values
- When need to refer to a specialty physician, a nurse practitioner, a psychologist, a surgeon, or an HIV specialist, select one who is a trans-competent professional[6]
- Determine the severity of the patient's gender dysphoria-related distress, and thoroughly evaluate level of interest in future transgender hormonal therapy or surgery
- Monitor for increased risks for associated diseases in transgender individuals thinking of taking feminizing or masculinizing hormones
- For individuals with gender dysphoria:
  a) eliminate gender differential diagnoses, to include stress-relieving cross-dressing, sexual orientation issues, compulsive cross-dressing, gender confusion, and psychopathology[3]
  b) make a determination as to the adolescent's cross-dressing experiences, fantasies, and expectations; the extreme challenges that sex reassignment may bring as well as its potential benefits
  c) psychotherapy is essential for transgender youth

Gender Dysphoria Problems

prior to sex reassignment surgery; individual alone or combined with group therapy are supportive and effective. Family therapy is also beneficial where conflict exists
- Among transgender youth who seek sex reassignment, three different expert viewpoints for hormone therapy exist: a) No hormones before legal age of consent (usually age 18); b) adolescents should experience puberty to at least Tanner 4 or 5 (15-16 years of age; and c) adolescents may be eligible for hormonal suppression of puberty after Tanner Stage 2 or 3, typically 12-13 years of age, if criteria fulfilled[7]
- An adolescent who presents for transition therapy or sex reassignment may have already begun the transition process him- or herself through hormones, and may already be cross-dressing or living life in the desired gender. In addition, during his or her childhood, he or she may have had marked GD and fear of puberty, so may have received hormonal therapy for suppression of puberty
- Discuss the criteria and implications of fully reversible interventions achieved by pubertal delay; partially reversible interventions achieved by feminizing and masculinizing hormones; and irreversible interventions through surgery[7]

- Ensure patient's understanding, acceptance, and commitment

Fully Reversible Interventions

- Psychotherapy is not required prior to beginning transgender endocrine therapy; however, an assessment by a mental health physician or nurse who is trans-competent for management of transgender endocrine therapy/transition is required[3]
- For approved adolescents, begin male growth hormones to delay or prevent further pubertal changes if desired and approved, and continue hormones and cross-living if previously initiated and committed

Partially Reversible Interventions

- Begin transgender endocrine therapy with the use of feminizing hormones for men who desire to become *their inner woman,* and masculinizing hormones for women who wish to become *their inner man*
- Implement the Real Life Experience (RLE) in which the person of transgender lives full-time in the role into which he or she is transitioning and adopts all activities of daily living associated with that role. A

person is expected to function for two years in the RLE before making the irreversible changes of surgery, and adolescents have to have experienced RLE since the age of 16 before surgery is considered[3]

Irreversible Interventions

- "Sex reassignment surgery refers to a number of procedures that can be undertaken to surgically feminize or masculinize the face, neck, breasts or chest, genitals, and overall body contours; stop menstrual periods (FTM); raise voice pitch (MTF)"[7(p26)]
- Adolescents must have a mental health evaluation and support prior to and during surgical transition
- The cost of the many surgeries associated with transition surgery often precludes the person of transgender bodily transitioning into his or her desired sex as few insurance companies reimburse

F. Supportive Interventions

- Review the Supportive Interventions Guide for Adults (Appendix H)
- Perform a modified sexual assessment
- Determine any prior attempts of feminizing or

masculinizing to achieve body and gender congruence through unconventional or conventional means
- Determine how the patient thinks and feels about being transgender, how it has impacted relational aspects of his or her life (family, friends, partner), and what are his or her support networks; employment, finances (many persons of transgender live in poverty), housing status, and available health benefits; and self-worth, self-esteem, presence of depression, self-harm, or suicidal ideation or suicide attempt, among others
- Provide sexual education, preoperative/postoperative teaching, teaching for HIV/STI prevention or treatment
- Provide support and education about body image changes, and refer for hair removal, suitable attire, hair/wigs; mannerisms, walking, body positioning, and voice
- Obtain social service referral to assist patient's application for needed benefits such as health, housing, food stamps, allowances, pensions, etc.
- Support and educate the adolescent and adult when he or she has decided to *come out* as being transgender and transitioning
- Explain the procedures associated with the actual reassignment surgery and the expectations for post-operative care
- Perform all aspects of post-operative care

G. Potential Outcomes

- In their follow-up study of 77 children, 59 boys and 18 girls, (average age 18 plus years), Wallien and Cohen-Kettenis[7] found that 12 boys and 8 girls still identified after puberty as having GID (*persistence* group). Nearly all the males and females in this group identified as being homosexual or bisexual. Of those in the *desistence* group, all the girls and half the boys identified as being heterosexual, while the other half of the boys identified as being homosexual or bisexual. Most become comfortable with their natal gender over time, and are classified in the desistence group
- This small group of children become adults who will choose to do one of a few things: nothing at all, cross-dress into their desired sex, take hormonal therapy to change to their desired sex without transition surgery, or take hormonal therapy and transition surgery to change to their desired sex[7]

Points for Discussion:

How would you approach discussion of the outcomes of this study with the parents of a child who demonstrates symptoms of gender dysphoria?

SECTION 5

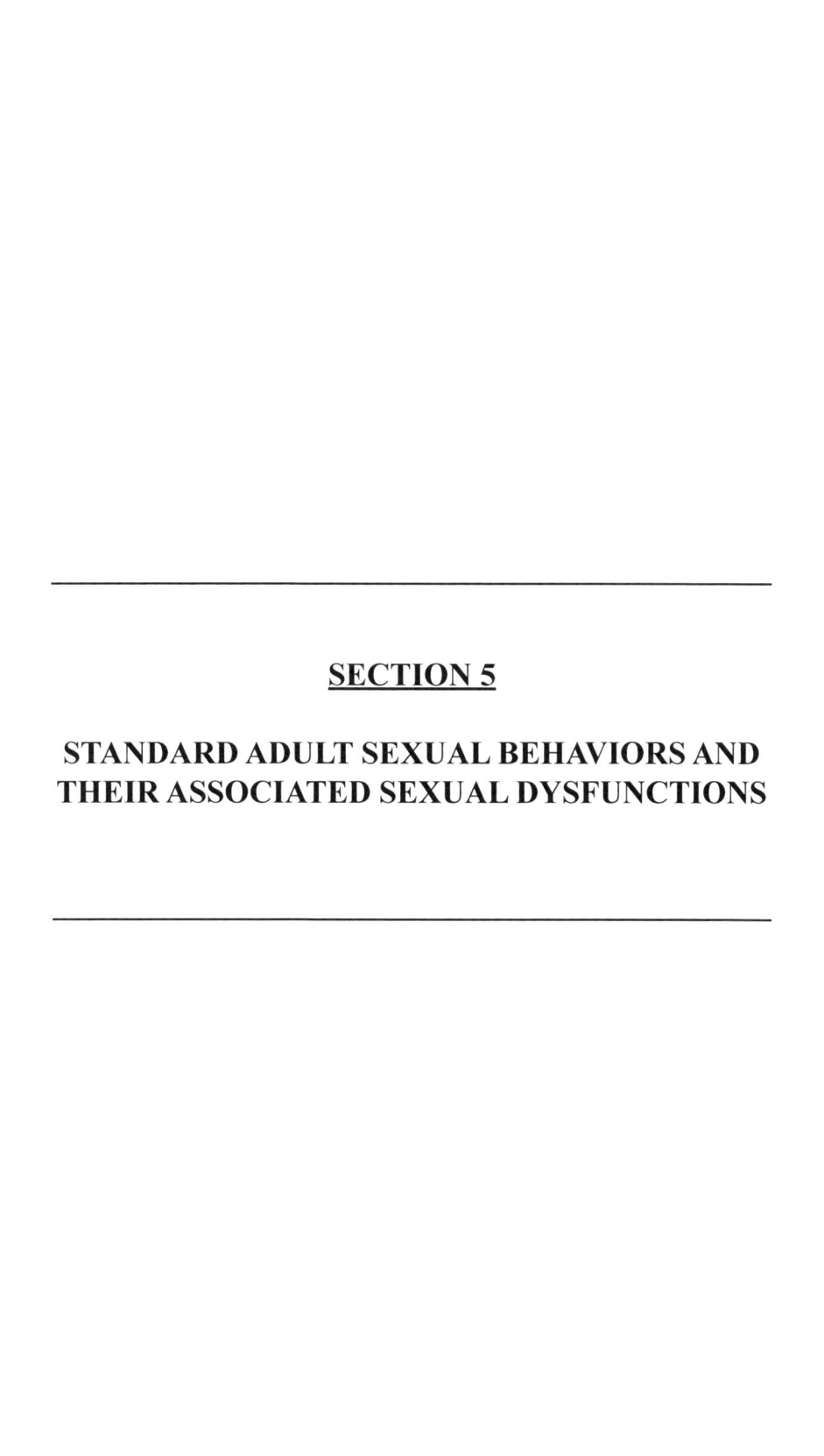

STANDARD ADULT SEXUAL BEHAVIORS AND THEIR ASSOCIATED SEXUAL DYSFUNCTIONS

CHAPTER 8

SEXUAL DYSFUNCTIONS IN MEN AND WOMEN AND THE LEARNED BEHAVIORS THAT CONTRIBUTE TO THOSE DYSFUNCTIONS

"A very large majority of men and women in America feel loved, feel satisfied, even thrilled by their sex partners, and that comparatively few are made to feel sad, or afraid, or guilty. Nevertheless, there are many specific problems that can arise in connection with sexual activity."

— Edward O. Laumann, Sex Researcher

Sexual behavior problems in American adults are classified for convenience into three general categories, which are frequently used to begin discussions about adult sexual concerns. These three categories are: 1. Sexual dysfunctions, 2. Gender identity and gender development concerns, and 3. Paraphilias.

1. **Sexual Dysfunctions** are an alteration in one or more of the first three phases of the four-part human sexual response cycle (desire, arousal, orgasm, resolution) as a result of psychological, physiological, or combined causes. Mental health professionals have categorized these dysfunctions into sub-types: lifelong or acquired, generalized, or situational. Researchers have found sexual dysfunctions to be highly prevalent in America. They affect 43% of women and 31% of men, with premature ejaculation the most frequent issue for men (30%), and desire disorders the most frequent issue for women (33%).[1] Sexual dysfunctions include the following conditions:

   A. Sexual Desire Disorders
      i. Low sexual desire disorder (hypophilia) in men
      ii. Low sexual desire disorder (hypophilia) in women
      iii. High sexual desire disorder (hyperphilia) in men
      iv. High sexual desire disorder (hyperphilia) in men
   B. Sexual Arousal Disorders
      i. Male erectile disorder
      ii. Female sexual arousal/lubrication disorder
   C. Orgasm Disorders in Men and Women
      i. Female orgasm disorder (FOD)
      ii. Male orgasm disorder (MOD)
   D. Ejaculation disorders in men and lubrication disorders in women

i. Ejaculation disorders in men
   ii. Lubrication disorders in women
E. Sexual Pain Disorders in Men and Women
   i) Vulvodynia in women
   ii) Vaginismus in women
   iii) Dyspareunia in women
   iv) Dyspareunia in men

*"Sexual behavior has three components:
sexual capacity (what an individual can do sexually);
sexual motivation (what an individual wants to do sexually);
andsexual performance (what an individual
actually does do sexually)."*

— Lester A. Kirkendall

Learned Behaviors that Contribute to Sexual Behavior Problems in Adults

Specific factors contribute to learned behaviors that predispose a child or adolescent toward adult sexual behavior problems. Sexual problems can be biological, psychological, and physiological; may have a number of contributing factors; and can range from the simple to the complex.

Many sexologists, sex therapists, and psychologists believe that sexual behavior problems, especially sexual dysfunctions, are the result of behaviors learned during childhood and adolescence, and as such, these behaviors can be unlearned and changed. A number of factors contribute to learned sexual behaviors, including:

- Narrow religious beliefs and religiosity of the child's parents, together with a rigid upbringing with excessive discipline, especially punishment for masturbation
- Socio-economic upbringing and status within the community
- The child's level of education
- Sex is portrayed by culture, then perceived by some as *dirty and shameful*, an act done in the dark, with a partner's body often not seen
- Women who have lots of sex are referred to as *sluts* or *promiscuous*, while men who have lots of sex are *just having fun; boys will be boys*
- Sexual and cultural scripts and societal expectations within the community of a child's upbringing. A) Male sexual scripts such as male dominance, sex is primarily for male pleasure, assertiveness and aggression, and decision-making; male sexual intercourse initiation, the need for and acceptance of male visual sexual stimulation, multiple sexual encounters for men, and sexual prowess and performance. B) Female sexual scripts such as subservience and weakness, sexual compliance and obedience, with rare or minimal sexual initiation; less consideration for female sexual satisfaction, female sexual

passivity, resigned acceptance, that is begrudgingly and silently tolerated; procreation is the goal
- The societal sexualization of young children, especially young girls and female adolescents
- Sources of sex education for children and adolescents are varied; information is frequently inaccurate and misconstrued, and myths and inconsistencies abound
- Altered or deficient family communication patterns

Sexual dysfunctions may be lifelong, acquired, generalized or situational.

— DSM-3 psychiatrists

A) Sexual Desire Disorders
   i) **Low sexual desire disorder in men**

   a. **Definition.** Persistent, recurrent, absence of any sexual fantasies and desires for sexual activity in a man that results in severe distress or interpersonal difficulties for the individual and his partner.

   b. **Signs and Symptoms**

   - A man with a low sexual desire avoids any

opportunity for sex and demonstrates no interest in sex whatsoever. He does not touch or cuddle his partner outside or inside the bedroom from fear of partner perceiving it as a sexual invitation
- He does not initiate sex and has no fantasies or sexual thoughts whatsoever
- May withdraw from his partner verbally and physically
- Activities that used to stimulate him sexually no longer do
- Distressed as a result of perceived sexual failure that results in relationship issues with partner, and interpersonal and intrapersonal difficulties
- Complains that sex is boring, predictable, and lacks its prior spark, excitement, and newness

c. Origins

- Often associated with erection and/or orgasm issues that cause loss of self-esteem and a man's general sense of wellbeing
- Relationship issues with his longtime partner and non-availability of others as a man ages
- Chronic conditions such as arthritis, diabetes, hypertension, low thyroid, low testosterone,

and depression, and the adverse side effects of treatment medications, especially antidepressants in the serotonin reuptake inhibitors (SSRIs) category
- Excessive use of alcohol and illegal drugs such as heroin and cocaine
- Performance anxiety as the man fears partner or he will not climax, or he will prematurely ejaculate
- A discrepancy between a man and his partner's levels of sexual desire
- Has lost feelings for his partner, especially sexual feelings
- Exhaustion from work, taking care of children, financial issues; mundane life, boredom, and stress of day-to-day activities

d. Background

- Laumann et al.[1] found that 31% of men suffer from serious sexual issues, 15% of whom say they lack interest in sex, and 15% derive no pleasure from sex. Single men experience more lack of desire than married men, and 15.8% of men between ages of 15 and 59 have persistent

complaints of low sexual desire. Seven percent of men experience loss of sexual desire in their 20s, 12% in their 40s, 18% between 50 to 59, and in the 60s, there is a rise to 25 to 30%
- Loss of sexual desire impacts men more harshly than women; even if low desire is present for them, 46% of women are still happy about their lives, while only 23% of men are happy[1]

e. Therapeutic Interventions

- Perform Standard Sexual Assessment (Appendix C) and medical assessment, and obtain sexual and medical histories
- Discontinue any potential offending medications, such as SSRIs, and advise to discontinue use of illegal substances and alcohol, if a factor
- Evaluate the couple for relationship issues such as anger, frustration, denial, guilt, sadness, rejection, loneliness, motivation, and commitment or lack of commitment to relationship
- Implement couple therapy if indicated
- Implement psychotherapy if a conflict from prior sexual and physical abuse exists
- Implement cognitive behavioral therapy (CBT)

Sexual Dysfunctions

to provide cognitive restructuring about sex, to reduce avoidance of partner and sex, and to reduce overall anxiety
- Explain about Sensate Focus and its associated techniques (Sensate Focus is sex therapy to promote closeness and intimacy, the use of body touch rather than genital, and to relearn about own and partner's body likes and dislikes to increase intimacy and improve the quality and type of sexual activities; see also Appendix D)

f. Supportive Interventions

- Review the Supportive Interventions Guide for Adults (Appendix H)
- Perform physical and sexual assessment and obtain past and current sexual history
- Evaluate couple's level of sexual knowledge and understanding; discuss potential sexual dysfunction, and potential treatments
- Reinforce the tender touch, tender talk, and tender thoughts associated with Sensate Focus (Appendix D)
- Evaluate couple's relationship, their commitment to the relationship, and communication, and relationship skills; support them during couple therapy and CBT

- Teach relaxation and breathing techniques, as well as body image exercises, positive self-esteem exercises
- Encourage the couple to exercise; explore new interests; go out with friends (will see partner in different light); discuss courting techniques such as dates, watch romantic, fun films together; then move to more sexually *provocative* ones as progress is made

g. Potential Outcomes

- If the therapy is maintained and adhered to, low sexual desire issues may be somewhat alleviated, although if interpersonal relationship and emotional issues continue, a positive outcome is unlikely
- Relapse is possible if precipitating/contributing factors persist or reoccur
- A highly motivated man and the continued involvement of a partner achieve better outcomes

ii) Low sexual desire disorder in women

a. **Definition.** Persistent, recurrent, or absence of any sexual fantasies or desire for sexual activity in a woman that results in severe distress or interpersonal and intrapersonal difficulties for the individual and her partner

b. Signs and Symptoms

- A woman persistently lacks interest in any form of sexual expression, including sensuality, erotica, sexual thoughts and fantasy, sexual touch, emotional intimacy. She rarely (if ever) initiates sex, and if she does, she does so unwillingly and grudgingly
- Frequently combined with other sexual issues such as lack of arousal, orgasmic disorder, or painful sexual intercourse (dyspareunia)
- In the bedroom, the woman is acutely aware of non-sexual extraneous items and activities as well as sexual interruptions that interfere with any emergence of desire for her partner—children or mother-in-law overhearing, interruptions, fears of STIs or pregnancy, changed body and genital image, self-image, etc. But, most importantly, her positive or negative feelings toward her partner and their present level of intimacy and wellbeing determine the amount of desire she feels, how receptive she is, and how much she wants and decides to participate[2]

c. Origins

- Origins can be physical, psychological, or emotional; lifelong, acquired, generalized, or situational
- Obtain a medical and standard sexual history "…include three factors that contribute to sexual dysfunction: past psychosexual development, current life context; and medical factors, including comorbid illness, drugs and previous surgery"[2]
- Many potential contributing factors of everyday life include fatigue, too busy, misunderstandings, hurt feelings, family-related issues, child-bearing and rearing, adultery, work-related issues, financial problems, and past and present sexual abuse
- Relationship issues that lead to feelings of inadequacy, resentment, apathy, or anger
- Low self-esteem, poor self-image, and poor physical and emotional health
- Rigid upbringing, the type of culture in which raised, religious orthodoxy or religiosity in the family and lack of accurate sexual knowledge
- Overemphasis by partner on genitalia, coitus,

orgasm, maximum performance, and male initiation
- A low desire for sex seen in chronic medical conditions such as diabetes, heart disease, and low estrogen levels; depression especially is strongly associated with a low desire for sex
- Excess ingestion of medications and substances such as opioids, antidepressants, anti-hypertensives, anxiolytics, sedatives, and hypnotics
- Reduction in woman's estrogen and testosterone levels, especially with advancing age

d. Background

Laumann[1] and his colleagues found that:
- 33% of women experience a lack of interest or desire at some point in their lives; 10% or less of the population below age 50 have not had sex in the past year, and only 20% or less report having sex a few times a year to monthly under age 40
- 43% of women suffer from serious sexual issues, with lack of interest being the most common; 32% of women admit that they

seldom want sex, 27% state they do not enjoy sex, and 26% report sexual anxiety
- Sexual problems are highest among women ages 18-29, especially single women
- 42% of female high school dropouts report a lack of desire, compared to 24% of female college students[1]
- The person with low sexual desire, either man or woman, controls the sexual relationship

e. Therapeutic Interventions

- Perform a Standard Sexual Assessment (Appendix C) and a medical assessment, and obtain a sexual and medical history
- Interventions are similar to low sexual desire in men
- Discontinue any potential offending medications and advise to discontinue use of illegal substances and alcohol, if a factor
- Evaluate the couple for relationship issues such as anger, frustration, denial, guilt, sadness; rejection, loneliness, motivation, and commitment or lack of commitment to the relationship

- Implement couple therapy if needed. Medical practitioner implements specific treatments according to his or her expertise, experience, previous successes, and specific contributing factors
- Types of therapies include behavior therapy, cognitive-behavioral therapy, couple therapy, fantasy therapy, psychoanalytical therapy, bibliotherapy, Sensate Focus, and biomedical therapy (Appendix D)

f. Supportive Interventions

- Review the Supportive Interventions Guide for Adults (Appendix H)
- Obtain sexual and medical history, actively listen to person's description of sexual desire issues, and assess precipitating factors in need of reduction
- Discuss the treatment plan and evaluate understanding and commitment
- Implement identified therapeutic approach, evaluate results, and modify if needed
- Assign exercises and educate/demonstrate

techniques (e.g., intimacy techniques, Kegel exercises, relaxation techniques, massage techniques, Sensate Focus techniques, etc.).
- Evaluate sexual knowledge accuracy, provide remediation for inaccuracies, and refer to sex therapist if indicated
- Obtain and administer medications such as anxiolytics, hormones, relaxants; equipment or supplies needed for the planned interventions
- Support individual in degree of effort and achievements and acknowledge failure

g. Potential Outcomes

- If the therapy continues and is adhered to, low sexual desire issues may be somewhat alleviated, although if interpersonal/relationship and emotional issues persist, a positive outcome is unlikely
- A highly motivated woman and continued involvement of the partner achieve better outcomes
- Relapse is possible if precipitating/contributing factors persist or reoccur

B. Sexual Arousal Disorders

i. Male erectile disorder (ED)

a. Definition. A man's inability to have a penile erection or to maintain an erection that is firm enough for partner-related sexual activities, especially sexual intercourse or anal or oral sex to the satisfaction of the man and or his partner. Other sexual issues may or may not be present.

b. Signs and Symptoms

- Persistence of a non-erect, limp penis, which the man is unable to insert into a partner's vaginal or anal orifice or mouth, or loss of tumescence during penetration or thrusting
- Exhibited or verbalized distress by the man or his partner, as well as a reduction in sexual desire
- As the man's ED persists, his anxiety rises, and as his anxiety rises, the ED worsens
- Evidence of increased interpersonal sexual and relationship issues between man and partner

c. **Origins**

- Three biological functions must work efficiently before normal erectile function can take place—the nerve supply, the blood supply, and the brain supply—and any interference in one impacts overall erectile function
- Primary origins are physical and related to a) blood vessel disease, to include atherosclerosis, high blood pressure, heart disease, diabetes, and tobacco use; b) hormonal and metabolic disease, to include low testosterone, high cholesterol, and high insulin levels; and c) diseases to include Parkinson's disease, multiple sclerosis, and Peyronie's disease.[3] Secondary origins are psychological and occur as a result of ED, to include emotional distress, depression, increased anxiety, mental health conditions, alcohol and drug abuse
- Other important origins include relationship issues, sexual performance anxiety, continued pressure on the pelvic nerves (as in bicycling), pressure on the spinal cord, genitalia trauma and surgery, fragile relationship with sex partner, fatigue, and poor physical health

Sexual Dysfunctions

d. Background

- ED is a common condition, and its prevalence increases with advancing age
- Single men experience more ED than married men, and many men experience great distress as a direct result of ED
- ED may sometimes serve as a lifeline for both partners, such as for the man who does not want sex with his partner, and for the partner who is relieved not to have to have sex

e. Therapeutic Interventions

- Perform a Standard Sexual Assessment (Appendix C) and medical assessment, and obtain a sexual and medical history
- Determine blood levels to indicate any risk factors for a chronic disorder. Disorders such as elevated lipids, kidney disease, low hematocrit and sex hormone deficiency levels
- Advise patient to reduce stress, blood pressure, and smoking; relax more, sleep more, and talk with his partner more
- Ultrasound to measure blood flow and a venous

- leak, nocturnal tumescence (normal six erections nightly), arteriography, among others
- Effective treatments are sex counseling, especially cognitive-behavioral therapy, as well as Viagra, Cialis, and Levitra, and a supportive, understanding partner
- Other treatments include alprostadil as an intracavernosal penile injection and pellets into the urethra, vacuum constrictive devices (not well-received by patients), and prostaglandin cream to the tip of penis
- Sensate Focus
- Sex therapy by sex therapist or sexologist

f. **Supportive Interventions**

- Review Supportive Interventions Guide for Adults (Appendix H)
- Discuss ED with male and partner, identify potential precipitating factors
- Explain about diagnostic tests needed to diagnose or confirm ED, treatments, and possible favorable outcomes
- Explain, demonstrate, and support patient during penile injections, vacuum devices, pellet insertion, etc.

Sexual Dysfunctions

- Educate about the risk factors associated with ED, to include drug and alcohol use and use of antihypertensives, antihistamines, and muscle relaxants; and diuretics, hormones, chemotherapy, and antidepressants
- Discuss the effects of obesity, diabetes, elevated stress levels on ED, and resulting anxiety and depression
- Assess patient understanding of those risk factors and patient's commitment to their prevention
- Educate about side effects of Cialis, Levitra, and Viagra, such as headaches, flushing, indigestion, severe hypotension (if taken with nitrates), and potential for prolonged erections (priapism)
- Explain the steps, exercises, and expectations of Sensate Focus
- Encourage the completion of assignments—reading, exercises such as intimacy building—to increase sensuality, improve interpersonal dynamics, reduce anxiety, reduce penile and genital preoccupation

g. **Potential Outcomes**

- Viagra, Levitra, and Cialis do not cure relationship

Understanding Patients' Sexual Problems

issues or sexual problems or eradicate sexual difficulties. They do, however, provide a favorable outcome to the penile erection issue by usually resulting in a sustained erection
- Sexual therapy is most helpful if a man can have normal erections during sleep, if he complies with assignments/treatments and does not discontinue after just a few sessions
- ED may not be an ongoing issue for the man and his partner since it may resolve spontaneously

ii. **Female sexual arousal disorder (FSAD) (or vaginal lubrication disorder)**

  a. **Definition.** The persistent and recurring inability of a woman to attain and maintain sexual excitement that results in vaginal and genital lubrication and engorgement. Basson et al.[2] identified five sub-types to include generalized arousal disorder, genital arousal disorder, mixed arousal disorder, dysphoric arousal disorder, and anhedonic arousal disorder. The condition can be lifelong, acquired, situational, or generalized

  b. **Signs and Symptoms**
     - Absence of vaginal/genital lubrication, and of smooth

Sexual Dysfunctions

   muscle relaxation
- Painful intercourse due to dry vagina
- Evidence of distress due to disappointment and relationship issues

c. Origins

- Past psychosocial and psychosexual development, current life situation, and medical conditions such as diabetes mellitus and diabetic neuropathy, multiple sclerosis, heart, liver, or kidney disease; pelvic injury, spinal cord injury, illicit drugs, alcohol, and prescribed medications, especially SSRIs
- Insufficient foreplay, lack of clitoral stimulation, emotionally removed or emotionally distressed with partner
- Depression is a major contributor, as is absence of emotional intimacy with partner
- Learned sexual behaviors based on folklore, myths, misconceptions, culture, upbringing, etc.
- Woman is not aroused by her partner's efforts because of extraneous situational circumstances such as lack of privacy, fear of unwanted pregnancy, fear of an STI, and poor self-image; performance anxiety; disinterest in, boredom with, or fear of

partner; and concerns about body imperfections that distract her during preliminary sexual activities[2]
- Post-menopausal lubrication reduction due to hormonal changes

d. **Background**

- Effects about 20% of women, especially younger women
- Sexual problems of women usually diminish with age, but not arousal disorder
- Women of different racial groups demonstrate different presentations of sexual dysfunctions, Hispanic women experience fewer problems with arousal disorder than Caucasian and African-American women
- Often accompanied by other sexual dysfunctions such as desire and orgasmic issues

e. **Therapeutic Interventions**

- Perform a Standard Sexual Assessment (Appendix C) and medical assessment, and obtain sexual and medical histories
- Refer to psychologist, sex therapist, or psychiatric

nurse practitioner; general nurses may also be involved
- Implement Cognitive Behavioral Therapy, bibliotherapy, and clitoral masturbation therapy
- Bibliotherapy is especially helpful for women; men respond to visual erotica while women respond to sexual stories
- Medications to include anxiolytics and antidepressants
- Reduction of relationship issues with partner, especially with couple therapy and Sensate Focus to include self and partner calming and pleasuring
- Reduction of cognitive distortions that may be present
- Avoid Viagra-like medications as they are unsuccessful in women

f. **Supportive Interventions**

- Review the Supportive Interventions Guide for Adults (Appendix H)
- Obtain social services support and financial services support to alleviate family and life stressors
- Discussion of contributing factors and circumstances such as boredom, disgust, and/or dislike of her partner, his body and breath odors, lack of cleanliness, his sexual techniques, as well as others that may be frightening or make her

anxious to address with her partner
- Encourage the completion of all assignments and exercises, especially clitoral masturbation and bibliotherapy
- Describe and demonstrate Sensate Focus

g. Potential Outcomes

- Treatment of FSAD is often successful and frequently lasting; however, without therapy or elimination of the contributors, often continued distress and relationship issues exist for a woman and her partner

"The anthropologist Margaret Mead concluded in 1948, after observing seven different ethnic groups in the Pacific Islands, that different cultures made different forms of female sexual experience seem normal and desirable. The capacity for orgasm in women, she found, is a learned response which a given culture can help or fail to help its women to develop. Mead believed that a woman's sexual fulfillment and the positive meaning of her sexuality in her own mind, depend upon three factors:

1. She must live in a culture that recognizes female desire as being of value;

*2. Her culture must allow her to
understand her anatomy;
3. And her culture must teach the various
sexual skills that give a woman orgasms."*

— Naomi Wolf

C. Orgasm and Ejaculation Disorders

i) Female orgasm disorders

Female orgasm disorders include primary anorgasmia (never experienced an orgasm), and secondary (previously experienced orgasm) not now experiencing, even though using previously effective methods for orgasm achievement; situational (achieved in one setting but not another, with one particular person but not another), or generalized (always—wherever, whenever, with whomever)

    a. **Definition.** Orgasm is an extremely pleasurable response to sexual behavior brought about by a combination of many biological, physiological, and psychological factors. Any interference in the actions of one or more of these factors during the orgasm process can result in a disorder in orgasm

b. **Signs and Symptoms**
   - A woman's persistent inability to achieve orgasm, even though she wants to orgasm, is adequately stimulated and is sexually aroused
   - Marked distress in the woman about her inability to orgasm that brings about depression and may result in relationship issues with her partner

c. **Origins**
   - Psychological factors such as low self-esteem, poor body and genital image, relationship issues (especially intimacy), lack of confidence sexually, and ineffective communication with partner
   - Medical conditions such as diabetes and associated neuropathy, liver and kidney disease, atherosclerosis, spinal cord injuries, pelvic trauma, and alcohol and drug abuse
   - Drugs such as SSRIs as well as illegal drug abuse
   - Menopausal hormonal changes contribute to anorgasmia in women
   - Interpersonal factors are primary reasons for sexual dissatisfaction, such as her partner's hygiene, unacceptable or unusual sexual demands, perceived excessive frequency of sexual demands; dislike of and lack of attraction

to partner; unhappy with his or her appearance, poor hygiene, poor manners, and overall attitude of partner, among others

d. Background
- Some women have never experienced an orgasm, some rarely, some may need to be alone to do so, and some only orgasm with the use of a vibrator. In some women, the orgasm may be clitoral, vaginal, during coitus with other than vaginal stimulation, and result from erotic-associated activities that include fantasizing, talking dirty, massage, visual stimulation, erotic books, videos, etc.
- Anorgasmia occurs far more frequently in women than men
- Anorgasmia is the second most frequent sexual complaint of women, especially with vaginal intercourse alone. Clitoral stimulation is the most effective way for a woman to achieve orgasm; however, men usually expect women to achieve orgasm via vaginal intercourse
- Difficulty achieving orgasm for women occurs less frequently with age and being married

e. **Therapeutic Interventions**
- Perform a Standard Sexual Assessment (Appendix C) and medical assessment and obtain sexual and medical histories
- Involve other experts such as a psychologist, psychiatrist, or sexologist, a mental health nurse practitioner, and a physiotherapist
- Implement Cognitive Behavioral Therapy to promote positive changes in the woman's attitude toward herself generally as well as her sexual self, to alter positively her responses to her partner, to reduce sexual anxiety, and to identify any cognitive distortions about sex
- Couple therapy to address communication, relational, and interpersonal issues, as well as difficult to discuss topics such as her partner's personal hygiene, unacceptable type of sexual demands, and perceived excessive frequency of sexual demands
- Discuss and present an overall picture of Sensate Focus and its goals
- Psychological analysis (if psychological issues seem to be intense and deep-seated)
- Prescribe hormonal patches when woman's hormone levels indicate the need

Sexual Dysfunctions

- Describe and show videos of masturbation methods and internal and external vibrator use
- Prescribe Eros Clitoral handheld pump to increase blood flow of clitoris
- Physical therapy to strengthen woman's pelvic muscles
- Advise the woman to explore herself sexually and pleasure herself sexually as well as use of a vibrator (if her value-system permits)
- Reduce SSRI antidepressants if indicated

f. **Supportive Interventions**
- Review the Supportive Interventions Guide for Adults (Appendix H)
- Provide sex education about orgasms, positions and methods for achievement, together with masturbation techniques to include the Betty Dodson Method and use of the Hitachi Wand. Include her partner in the discussion, and assist both
- Determine what types of books are of interest, and suggest bibliotherapy as needed
- Identify and discuss interpersonal issues between woman and her partner, and determine interpersonal communication techniques that

would be successful
- Discuss the idiosyncrasies of her partner that contribute to woman's attitude toward her partner such as her appearance, attitude, partner's hygiene, manners, actions, etc., and discuss alternative ways to respond and address these issues. Discussion of these sensitive issues are often difficult for a woman to share
- Teach Kegel (pubococcygeus/pelvic) muscle exercises
- Describe steps and progression of Sensate Focus

g. **Potential Outcomes**
- Use of the Hitachi Wand, Betty Dodson masturbation techniques, and general masturbation techniques have very positive outcomes, with over 93% success reported in a Danish study
- Most women who complete therapy can revisit their sexual selves, change their distorted sexual perceptions, achieve orgasm, and attain sexually satisfying lives
- Viagra and similar medications have not been demonstrated to be effective for the treatment of sexual dysfunctions in women

Sexual Dysfunctions

ii) Male orgasm disorders (MOD)

These disorders include primary anorgasmia (never experienced an orgasm), and secondary (previously experienced orgasm, but not experiencing now), even though using previously effective methods for orgasm achievement; situational (achieved in one setting but not another, with one particular person but not another), or generalized (always—wherever, whenever, and with whomever).

a. **Definition.** A type of sexual dysfunction in which a person cannot achieve orgasm, even with adequate stimulation. Far more common in women than in men.[4]

b. **Signs and Symptoms**
- Complaints of delayed orgasm; orgasm that is decreased in intensity, duration, and sexual pleasure; or an absence of orgasm. The lack of an orgasm results in sexual dissatisfaction and distress for the man and his partner
- Sexual performance anxiety, depression, avoidance of sexual activities, and uncomfortable atmosphere between the two partners
- Relationship issues with partner almost invariably follow

c. **Origins**
- Retrograde (backward) ejaculation of semen is often misdiagnosed as anorgasmia
- Reduced testosterone induces anorgasmia

d. **Background**
- Reaching orgasm is the expected culmination of sexual activities for men, unlike women in whom anorgasmia is a greater issue and occurs more often
- MOD is not a common complaint for which men seek advice and may occur once in a man's lifetime or never. When it does take place, it causes the man and his partner distress

e. **Therapeutic Interventions**
- Perform a Standard Sexual Assessment (Appendix C) and medical assessment, and obtain sexual and medical histories
- Involve a psychiatrist, psychologist, or sex therapist; psychiatric nurse practitioner
- Determine mode of therapy, either individual or group, of Cognitive Behavioral Therapy to promote positive changes in the man's attitude toward himself as well as his sexual self

- Reduce depression and anxiety, to alter positively his responses to his partner, and identify any cognitive distortions about sex
- Couple therapy to address communication, relational, and interpersonal issues
- Psychological analysis (if psychological issues seem to be intense and deep-seated)
- Prescribe testosterone if man's level is low, and rule out retrograde ejaculation
- Reduce or eliminate all offending medications, especially SSRIs, and prescribe an alternative

f. Supportive Interventions
- Review the Supportive Interventions Guide for Adults (Appendix H)
- Identify and discuss interpersonal issues between man and his partner, and determine interpersonal communication techniques that might prove successful. This is a difficult area as the reasons for the absent or delayed orgasm may be extremely personal for the man and difficult for him to verbalize
- Discuss the idiosyncrasies of the partner that may contribute to the man's attitude toward his partner such as his lack of attraction toward his partner, his

partner's hygiene, manners, appearance, behavior, views, etc., and discuss alternative ways to respond to them
- Rule out retrograde ejaculation by observation for the presence of sperm in the man's urine

g. Potential Outcomes
Specific outcomes unknown as the majority of men who experience this disorder do not usually mention the presence of anorgasmia or delayed orgasm

D. Ejaculation disorders in men and lubrication disorder in women

i. Male premature ejaculation

a. Definition. Premature ejaculation (PE) that occurs in men after minimal penile stimulation prior to intercourse, and occurs prematurely, either before, at, or just after vaginal or anal penetration, but always before both partners desire. The result is that neither the man nor his partner achieve sexual satisfaction

b. Signs and Symptoms
- Male and his partner express distress and concern with the prematurity of ejaculation

Sexual Dysfunctions

- Persistent and recurrent bouts of premature ejaculation occur during first thrusts of sexual intercourse
- Man may have feelings of sexual inadequacy for *letting his partner down*; with guilt, low self-esteem, and difficult intrapersonal relationships with his partner, as well as interpersonal difficulties with others
- May have marked distress if the situation is prolonged and relationship may be damaged

c. **Origins**
- Chronic medical conditions such as prostate infections and enlargement, urethritis, diabetes mellitus, atherosclerosis, among others
- Masturbation or sexual intercourse that was rushed when young, ejaculated quickly, with residual guilt
- Anxiety associated with early episodes of intercourse when young and inexperienced
- Excess guilt if premarital or extramarital intercourse, especially if has religious beliefs that contradict
- Possible hereditary component
- Infrequent sexual intercourse
- Fears of STIs, unwanted pregnancy

d. Background
- PE is the most frequently occurring sexual dysfunction in men, and prevalence varies widely, from less than 5% to greater than 40%.[5] The highest incidence is among men over age 60, but PE occurs in men of all ages
- PE causes a high rate of psychosocial distress, as well as interpersonal relationship issues with the man's sexual partner
- PE reduces the chances of sperm insemination and, consequently, impregnation, as well as reduces the opportunities for sexual pleasure

e. Therapeutic Interventions
- Routine assessment for medical conditions, infections of genitals, prostate, and urinary tract; treat any disorders that require interventions
- Prescribe tricyclic antidepressants, topical anesthetic to man's penis (although not appealing for partner), selective serotonin reuptake inhibitors (SSRIs)
- Determine and discuss therapeutic options to include couple therapy, prohibit intercourse for at least two weeks, Sensate Focus (especially if he has a supportive partner), must regain sexual intimacy for best effect; implement start-stop technique, and

squeeze technique
- Advocate masturbation for young men prior to next sexual intercourse, use of condoms, or with his partner on top

f. Supportive Interventions
- Review Supportive Interventions Guide for Adults (Appendix H)
- Examine relationship issues with patient and his partner
- Educate about the ejaculation process, discuss potential breakdown causes within that process, and discuss high possibility for success, and the planned interventions
- Demonstrate start-stop technique, squeeze technique, and discuss/demonstrate Sensate Focus
- Ensure compliance with medications and exercises through ongoing follow-up
- Emphasize the importance of a supportive partner and active involvement in the process
- Encourage open discussion about patient's sexual condition, treatment plan, and prognosis
- Evaluate for improved mood, involvement in Sensate Focus, intimacy achievement, etc.

g. **Potential Outcomes**
    - PE is one of the most successfully treated sexual conditions, especially with a caring, supportive partner. Success rate of treatment is stated by many to be 90% (Masters and Johnson claimed 99%)
    - If medications, Sensate Focus, and exercises are discontinued, or if supportive person withdraws from the relationship, any positive gains are frequently lost

"Sex is as important as eating or drinking and we ought to allow the one appetite to be as satisfied with as little restraint of false modesty as the other."

— Marquis de Sade

ii. **Absent ejaculation (anejaculation)**

a. **Definition.** A man's failure to ejaculate semen naturally, or with stimulation of the penis through intercourse or masturbation and stimulation. May be complete or situational according to the etiology.

b. **Signs and Symptoms**
    - An absence of ejaculate following adequate

stimulation of the penis
- Situational absence of ejaculation accompanied by evidence of distress; however, is usually able to have nocturnal emissions
- Some men may have anorgasmic anejaculation, others orgasmic anejaculation

c. **Origins**
- Psychological origins where a stressor causes the absence of ejaculation (situational)
- Transurethral resection or post prostate, bladder, and testicular cancer surgery result in no ejaculation and no orgasm (anejaculation and anorgasmia)[6]
- Prostate problems and post prostate or urethral surgery, bladder and testicular cancer, radiation therapy and nerve damage, diabetic neuropathy, MS, and spinal cord injury[6]
- Semen movement into the urethra from the prostate and seminal ducts is interrupted
- SSRIs may cause ejaculation without orgasm and anejaculation[6]

d. **Background**
- Some men may have an orgasm without ejaculation while others may ejaculate without orgasm

- Men who sustained complete or partial spinal cord injury do not ejaculate or orgasm

e. Therapeutic Interventions
- Perform a Standard Sexual Assessment (Appendix C) and medical assessment, and obtain a sexual and medical history
- CBT for situational symptoms, or refer to a sexologist or sex therapist if further sex therapy needed
- Vibrator therapy for extended stimulation to assist in sperm retrieval for insemination
- Discontinue offending SSRIs for men without spinal cord injuries, diabetes mellitus, or multiple sclerosis

f. Supportive Interventions
- Review the Supportive Interventions Guide for Adults (Appendix H)
- Assess psychosexual aspects and provide support
- Educate the patient about the anatomy and physiology of the urogenital system
- Support discussion about the man and his partner's desire to retrieve sperm for insemination, and assist with vibrator application sessions and sperm

collection
- Provide advice and support if interpersonal problems exist with the couple

g. **Potential Outcomes**
- Discontinuation of the SSIs usually ends the anejaculation problem if a spinal cord injury or multiple sclerosis not present
- Men with incomplete or complete spinal cord injury often lose the ability to have erections or reach orgasm
- Vibrator therapy helps 60% of men with anejaculation and spinal cord injury, which facilitates sperm retrieval for insemination directly into the uterus of the female partner [6]
- No treatment exists for successfully restoring ejaculation following prostate surgery

iii. **Retrograde ejaculation**

a. **Definition.** The complete absence of a forward moving ejaculate; a result of a backward flow of semen through the bladder neck into the bladder.

b. **Signs and Symptoms**

- Sperm is eliminated with passage of urine
- Man is unable to impregnate his female partner
- Dry orgasms

c. Origins
- Alpha blockers, antihypertensive medications, and mood-altering drugs
- Weakness of the bladder neck muscle and weak bladder neck permits sperm to enter the bladder instead of exiting via the urethra

d. Background
- Man may have psychological issues as a result of strict religious background that views sex as sinful
- Condition occurs infrequently and is usually harmless, although there is a chance of infertility
- Man may not be sexually attracted to his partner

e. Therapeutic Interventions
- Perform a Standard Sexual Assessment (Appendix C) and medical assessment, and obtain medical and sexual history
- Psychological consult if psychological issues present
- Post-ejaculation urinalysis to include screening for

semen in a man's urine that differentiates retrograde ejaculation from anejaculation
- Stop any offending medications and prescribe substitutions
- Implement imipramine and pseudo-ephedrine for closure of the bladder neck[7]

f. Supportive Interventions
- Review the Supportive Interventions Guide for Adults (Appendix H)
- Administer imipramine and pseudo-ephedrine for closure of the man's bladder neck
- Describe to patient how to screen and monitor his urine for the presence of semen
- Discuss any intrapersonal issues with the couple and seek expert assistance if unable to resolve

g. Potential Outcomes
- Administration of imipramine and pseudo-ephedrine usually manages the bladder neck issues
- Condition usually resolves if offending drugs discontinued

E. Sexual Pain Disorders including Vulvodynia in Women, Vaginismus in Women and Dyspareunia in Men and Women

i) Vulvodynia in women

    a. **Definition.** A chronic, painful condition of the vulva (labia, clitoris, and entrance to vagina) and lower part of the vagina; a multifactorial condition that challenges the health and wellbeing of the woman and her sexual partner

    b. **Signs and Symptoms**
- Severe pain within the vagina; a burning, searing, knifelike pain associated with burning, itching, and irritation of the vulva with stinging. Pain may be on touch, just around the vaginal entry (introitus) or generalized
- Not demonstrated to be related to time, situation, foods, or medications, but thought that there may be a stimulus or trigger of some kind
- Possible involvement of spasm of the pelvic floor muscles
- Vulval and vaginal erythema

    c. **Origins**
- True origin unknown, but may be associated with infections and associated inflammations such as candida, yeast, herpes, bladder-related, and vaginitis

- Irritants such as perfume, deodorants, douche solutions, soaps, clothing, etc.
- May be physical, psychological, sexual, or neurological in origin

d. Background
- Petersen et al.[8] demonstrate an incidence rate of 9-12% and may be as high as 18%
- Mostly in women 20-50 years old and those who are sexually active
- Difficult to diagnose, with no known cause or cure
- Not known to be related to STIs
- Chronic condition that makes life miserable for a woman and her partner

e. Therapeutic Interventions
- Perform a Standard Sexual Assessment (Appendix C) and medical assessment, and obtain a sexual and medical history
- Vulvodynia requires a combination of therapies rather than just one
- Obtain vaginal culture, and swab touch to determine whether there is an infection, to locate the pain, and identify potential irritants
- Evaluate pelvic floor muscles for spasms and tightness

- Prescribe anti-depressants, analgesics, and amitriptyline to reduce central nervous stimulation to vulva
- Estrogen creams for vaginal atrophy, local anesthetics, and biofeedback
- Implement physical therapy to provide pelvic floor exercises to strengthen muscles
- Administer Botox injections
- Perform laser ablation of vulval tissue
- Perform pudendal nerve block
- Refer for cognitive-behavioral therapy if indicated
- Advise comfort measures such as sitz baths, loose cotton underwear, water-based lubricants, analgesics

f. Supportive Interventions
- Review Supportive Interventions Guide for Adults (Appendix H)
- Determine the level of woman's pain and distress, educate about pain level identification, and use of analgesics
- Refer to a support group for women with vulvodynia; for example the National Vulvodynia Association[9]
- Demonstrate relaxation and self-soothing techniques to allay distress

- Educate about creams, vulval anesthetics, antibiotics, etc.
- Examine relationship issues and obtain a referral

g. **Potential Outcomes**
- Some women obtain relief if cause is identified or treatment effective; however, some do not, and condition may become chronic and difficult to manage
- Topical lidocaine and corticosteroidal creams have some effectiveness as does laser ablation of the vestibule
- Elimination of the offending organism or irritant affords the woman relief
- Cognitive-Behavioral Therapy may provide relief for anxiety, interpersonal, and sexual issues

ii) **Vaginismus**

a. **Definition.** A vaginal tightness causing discomfort, burning, pain, penetration problems, or complete inability to have intercourse.[10] May be primary or secondary

b. **Signs and Symptoms**
    - Involuntary muscle spasm of the muscles of the outer vaginal wall act as a rigid band or barrier that prevents insertion of a man's penis into the vagina; these spasms are beyond a woman's control
    - Muscle spasms cause the vaginal opening (introitus) to close so that nothing can be inserted, including a Tampon, fingers, partner's penis, speculum, etc.
    - Complaints of feelings of violation or invasion occur, not only of personal space but also of her body space if anything is inserted, often accompanied by fear and anxiety
    - Highly distressful for the woman, and often results in equally distressing relationship issues

c. **Origins**
    - Often occurs as a response to the anticipatory pain of dyspareunia; a self-protective mechanism
    - Woman possibly raised in an overly rigid, sexually negative home environment, with excessive religiosity; frequently with a domineering, overpowering father who may also have taken sexual advantage of his daughter. Or a woman's father may have been overly protective, and expected perfection in his daughter

- Medical conditions such as urinary tract infections, yeast infections, sexual trauma, and childbirth contribute to vaginismus
- Partner's sexual clumsiness or poor personal hygiene may be a factor
- Women in some cultures perceive sex to be *dirty, shameful, required, forced, not enjoyable, and barely tolerable*; these perceptions are passed down from a mother to her young daughter, who then develops her own less positive and even negative attitude toward sex
- Reduced vaginal lubrication
- Persistent fears of pregnancy, STIs, AIDs, and malignancy
- Experienced or witnessed past sexual abuse or trauma

d. **Background**
- Vaginismus is claimed to be 90% psychogenic and greater than 90% treatable
- No organic cause has been identified; however, genital surgery may contribute
- Roughly 2 in 1000 women have vaginismus,[10] although the true incidence is probably higher due to underreporting; a result of embarrassment, shame,

lack of education, fear, or improper diagnosis
- Some women may just live with the pain, or sexual relationships may go unconsummated
- Fear of sexual intercourse and insertion of her partner's penis causes the muscle tightening to increase, which then creates a repetitive vicious cycle
- Leads to avoidance of intimacy of any kind, and then loss of libido and any interest in sex

e. **Therapeutic Interventions**
- Discuss Kegel exercises to strengthen the vaginal muscles, encourage self-masturbation and body touching, and advise the woman to evaluate her own sexual anatomy and sexuality
- Vaginal desensitization with the use of graduated sized vaginal dilators; once dilated, partner may begin the gentle process of penile sexual intercourse
- Encourage to communicate with her partner as he attempts (very gradually and carefully) to insert his penis into his partner's vagina
- Sensate Focus exercises, massage, and gentle touch
- Prescribe anxiolytics, meditation exercises, relaxation techniques, and self-hypnosis for anxiety
- Botox injections into the muscles alongside the

vagina for the treatment of infrequent highly resistant vaginismus

f. Supportive Interventions
- Review Supportive Interventions Guide for Adults (Appendix H)
- Obtain a sexual history to help determine contributing factors
- Teach woman and partner about the woman's sexual anatomy and the contributing factors involved in vaginismus
- Teach patient tensing and relaxation exercises of the pelvic floor muscles
- Explain about the vaginal dilators, and assist woman and partner in the insertion of graduated vaginal dilators
- Explain goals and expectations of Sensate Focus and involved exercises and massage
- Discuss the intrapersonal situation between the woman and her partner and request a referral for psychological support if needed
- Teach about the efficacy of Botox injections and assist procedure as needed
- Self-hypnosis results have been promising

g. **Potential Outcomes**
   - Vaginismus has a high rate of treatability with success, greater than 90%
   - Interventions are mostly non-invasive and performed and controlled by the woman
   - If the contributing cause is removed and therapy adhered to and completed, the success usually lasts
   - Botox injections have been successful in the treatment of highly resistant vaginismus

iv. **Dyspareunia in women**

   a. **Definition.** Persistent and recurrent genital pain just before, during, or after intercourse. Painful intercourse can occur for a variety of reasons, ranging from structural problems to psychological concerns[11]

   b. **Signs and Symptoms**
   - Burning or aching pain at the entrance and within the woman's vagina at beginning, during, and after sexual intercourse; the pain becomes deeper within the pelvis, sometimes becomes unbearable with her partner's penile thrusting during sex
   - Relationship issues with partner due to pain anticipation and avoidance of intercourse

Sexual Dysfunctions

- Decreased or no interest in sex, satisfaction, and orgasm
- The woman may have a sex-negative orientation

c. **Origins**
- A result of factors that may be either physical, psychological, emotional, or cultural
- Genital and pelvic infections and trauma, insufficient vaginal lubrication (low estrogen with menopause, after childbirth, breastfeeding), post-episiotomy scarring, vaginismus, vulvodynia, uterine prolapse, retroverted uterus, hemorrhoids, pelvic infection disease, skin conditions, and infections[11]
- Medications that inhibit desire such as antidepressants, anti-hypertensives, antihistamines

d. **Background**
- Risk factors include sexual inexperience of one or both partners, and menopause and inadequate lubrication in the woman
- Higher incidence in women than men
- Patient may have a history of anxiety, poor self-image, and self-esteem issues, or the issues occur as a result of the dyspareunia
- May have intimacy and relationship issues with her

partner
- Stressed and depressed prior to, and/or related to dyspareunia

e. **Therapeutic Interventions**
- Obtain a standard sexual history and physical assessment, but usually unable to perform a pelvic examination with a speculum. Medical examination to include pelvic ultrasound/MRI to determine location of pain
- Determine whether woman has a history of sexual abuse, rape, or trauma; candida, herpes, genital warts, or other STIs
- Discuss any vaginal dryness, hot flushes, or menstrual symptoms
- Evaluate estrogen blood levels, especially if woman is menopausal
- Discontinue medications such as anti-hypertensives and antidepressants that may contribute to dyspareunia, and substitute others, if needed
- Discuss physical factors that contribute to dyspareunia to include infection, low estrogen levels, inadequate vaginal lubrication, and sequelae of pelvic surgery such as scarring, injury or trauma, radiation therapy, among others[12]

- Treatment is dependent upon the perceived origin of the dyspareunia to include antibiotics for infection, estrogen replacement for low estrogen, local corticosteroids, and vaginal lubricants for a low lubricant level
- Prescribe Kegel exercises to strengthen vaginal muscles
- Sex therapy and Sensate Focus as well as Cognitive Behavioral Therapy to increase intimacy, reduce fears, and improve intrapersonal relationship with her partner

f. **Supportive Interventions**
- Review Supportive Interventions Guide for Adults (Appendix H)
- Teach woman about her vaginal anatomy, explain potential location of the pain, and reinforce education about potential contributing factors
- Support the woman in her CBT therapy and activities to promote intimacy and improve intrapersonal relationship with her partner
- Encourage increase in foreplay to increase lubrication
- Discuss methods to raise a woman's feelings of self-worth and self-esteem

- Teach about the goals and processes of Kegel exercises and Sensate Focus
- Use of water-based lubricants before sex, wipe from front to back, sitz baths, urinate before and after intercourse

g. **Potential Outcomes**
- Treatment is usually long-term and may not always help[12]
- Psych-social causes often helped with therapy
- It is conveniently suggested that approximately one-third recover without treatment, one-third recover with treatment, and one-third continue to have pain and relationship issues

iv) **Dyspareunia in men**

a. **Definition.** Pain that occurs in a man's penis, his urethra, his pelvic region, or his perianal region before, during, or after sexual intercourse

b. **Signs and Symptoms**
- Pain in a man's penis, pelvic, or perianal area prior to, during, and after sexual intercourse
- Dyspareunia results in acute and chronic

Sexual Dysfunctions

embarrassment, distress, and discomfort with his situation, and he finds it difficult to discuss
- Associated signs and symptoms of the potential cause of the pain with intercourse
- Painful ejaculation at beginning probably due to penile urethral problem; after ejaculation, it is testicular in origin[13]

c. **Origins**
- Infections such as prostatitis, cystitis, and post-surgery, especially hernia repair
- Uncircumcised infection of the penis
- Antidepressants
- Skin disorders of the penis

d. **Background**
- Incidence is low, in the single digits[13]
- Dyspareunia in men is either underreported or occurs in a small percentage of men

e. **Therapeutic Interventions**
- Treatment of the perceived cause of the pain in men—vasculogenic, neurogenic, cystitis, psychological[13]

Understanding Patients' Sexual Problems

- Prescribe analgesics and antibiotics
- Administer tamsulosin for painful ejaculation/orgasm[14]

f. Supportive Interventions
- Review the Supportive Interventions Guide for Adults (Appendix H)
- Assist in pain management to include administration of analgesics, antibiotics, warm compresses, skin disease care
- Caution to abstain from intercourse until the primary cause eliminated
- Supportive therapy for man's embarrassment and distress

g. Potential Outcomes
- If the primary cause is eliminated, the pain will usually disappear; if not, the pain usually becomes chronic
- Tamsulosin is effective[14]

Points for Discussion:

Pat Morrison wrote (1/14/99) in the *Los Angeles Times*:
> The United States is sexually adolescent, simultaneously romantic and leering, marketing sex shamelessly in the service of capitalism, blushing and stammering about condoms and sex education until public policy is paralyzed. America is heterosexist, phallocentric, performance obsessed. The great taboos in America are sex, death, incest, and elimination.

What are your thoughts on this statement?

CHAPTER 9

SEXUALITY CONCERNS IN ADULTS THAT OCCUR AS A RESULT OF A CHRONIC ILLNESS, A SEVERE DISABILITY, AN END-OF-LIFE ILLNESS, OR OLDER AGE

"Dying people want to hear four very specific messages from their loved ones.
'Please forgive me, I forgive you, Thank you, I love you.'"

— Ira Byock

People with a disability, a chronic illness, or an end-of-life illness are the same as everybody else, with the same abilities, skills, and sexual needs and desires. They experience the same sexual dysfunctions and sexual disorders previously described. However, these individuals have the additional challenge of having a disease process that is frequently the cause of the sexual problems, and as the disease progresses, so do their sexual concerns. For the most part, the signs, symptoms, treatments, and potential outcomes are the same. However, additional barriers exist for patients in the treatment of sexual issues caused by the adverse sexual sequelae of their chronic or debilitating disease.

Healthcare professionals often regard a person with a chronic illness or disability as being devoid of thoughts of his or her sexuality as well as the sexuality of the partner; nothing could be further from the truth. The mind is often described as the body's greatest sexual organ, and in people with a chronic illness or disability, this statement is totally validated. Many people with these conditions have fulfilling fantasies, enjoy touch and intimacy, experience attraction and arousal, appreciate physical expressions of love and affection, and have desires and emotional relationships. They do, however, have to work harder to achieve them.

> *"Everyone has the right to experience their sexuality without fear of judgement. This is no less the case for people with dementia."*
>
> — Alzheimer's Society, 2012[1]

Alzheimer's Disease and Sexuality

A. Definition. A progressive, degenerative disorder that attacks the brain's nerve cells or neurons, resulting in loss of memory, thinking, and language skills, and behavioral changes.[2] The impact of Alzheimer's Disease on a person's sexuality and sex life varies from person to person, and partner to partner; it ranges from barely discernable to what some consider to be both life-changing and the end of their sex lives as previously known.

B. Signs and Symptoms
- "The person with Alzheimer's may have more interest in sex, less interest, or no interest in sex, more or less ability to perform sexually, changes in sexual 'manners' for example, appearing less sensitive to the other person's needs or appearing sexually aggressive, changes in levels of inhibitions (the person may say or do things that they would not have done previously"[1]
- The person with Alzheimer's experiences many losses—loss of role, companionship, understanding, communication, intimacy, love, involvement, and memories. These losses are replaced with a great need for love, affection, intimacy, affection, tenderness, touch, comfort, warmth, and communication, among others
- Sometimes one or both partners may feel varying degrees of upset, anger, loss, embarrassment, anxiety, or frustration, often in response to the patient's inappropriate behavior

- Inappropriate sexual behaviors include masturbation in front of others, touching another person's genitals, propositioning others, getting sexually aroused with another person not his partner, using obscene, offensive language, and stripping naked in front of other people
- Inappropriate sexual behaviors are usually not related to a need for sex at all; the patient may be too warm, wants to be comforted, hungry, wants to go to the bathroom, etc., but is unable to remember the right words
- Sometimes a patient does not recognize his partner, and confuses and assumes another person is his partner. May make sexual overtures or touch the person sexually in front of his partner
- The patient may have sexual intercourse and forget that it has ever taken place, much to the partner's dismay
- Perceived lack of cooperation by the partner to the patient's hypersexuality, and demands may lead to combative behavior by the patient against the partner

C. Origins
- Neurons produce the neurotransmitter acetylcholine (a messenger), which when they are damaged, break connections with other cells. Cells first degenerate in the hippocampus of the brain, which impacts short-term memory to the point that all short-term memory is lost.

Sexuality Concerns and Illness

Later, the cerebral cortex is affected, which results in language and judgment issues. All of these three losses impact sexuality—more or less interest in sex, more or less able to participate in sex, changes in levels of inhibitions, unpredictability, uses obscenities, and changes in sexual appropriateness. Unwelcome advances toward others are not intentional[2]
- Hypersexuality is usually the result of disinhibition (loss of control of inhibitions), the organic changes associated with aging, changes in relationship with partner to caregiver, and a loss of memory about what is socially acceptable; the patient just does not know his behavior is wrong
- Patient confusion is increased due to different surroundings, different rules, misinterpretation of cues (especially from television)

D. Background
- Alzheimer's disease is one type of dementia that usually occurs late in life, but it is also present in people below the age of 65
- Alzheimer's disease in one partner does not mean the end of the couple's sex life, although it usually manifests itself in a different form of physical contact that is more intimate, more peaceful, and more comfortable
- A person with dementia may form new and intimate

303

relationships that the grown children find hard to accept. They cannot believe their loved one still has sexual needs but for someone other than their parent who may or may not be deceased
- The patient and his/her partner may both withdraw sexually from the sexual relationship, and appear to be content to have that replaced with closeness, comfort, and intimacy[1]

E. Therapeutic Interventions
- Advise partner not to take any sexual withdrawal or aggression by his or her partner personally and always to maintain personal safety
- Inform partner that most incidents do not usually indicate a sexual meaning for the patient; rather, they are the result of other situations, such as patient confusion, patient's need for intimacy, for assurance of love, safety, closeness, and touch; a need to urinate, have a bowel movement, mistaken identity, etc.
- Educate partner to give his or her partner reassurance of safety, love, and caring, to avoid patient anger, and always try to provide a quiet, calm environment
- Inform partner to help the patient relieve sexual energy through exercise, masturbation, massage, music, singing, dance, etc.
- Refer to social worker or nurse specialist to provide partner

support and advice, or support groups of partners
- Medications are a last resort; however, when prescribed, include antipsychotics for delusions and aggression; antidepressants for irritability and depression; and anxiolytics for anxiety
- Use of a sex therapist is not usually indicated for persons with Alzheimer's, neither is the use of new and different alternative sexual activities helpful

F. Supportive Interventions
- Review the Supportive Interventions Guide for Adults (Appendix H)
- Educate the patient's partner and family about the disease process of Alzheimer's disease. When time is appropriate, prepare them for the future, without the use of *scare* tactics, excessive emotion, inaccurate information, or false hope
- Ensure the partner and family members are thoroughly educated about the impact that Alzheimer's disease has on their loved one, show them how to determine the cues their loved one gives that are associated with anxiety, pain, fatigue, etc. and the interventions to be made
- Advise partner about the use of touch, a soothing voice, increased intimacy and tenderness, and their effectiveness when intercourse is no longer an option
- Provide the caregiver with a list of resources for when the

Understanding Patients' Sexual Problems

patient's condition deteriorates
- Emphasize that the caregiver's safety and the safety of the loved one is paramount; teach methods to ensure that safety precautions are in place at all times
- Provide intervention guidelines for the partner of a person with Alzheimer's for when he or she behaves in a *sexually benign manner:*
    - Advise partner to accept masturbation or disrobing as a normal activity, and calmly take him to a different area to increase privacy
    - Focus on the person, not the behavior
    - Never ridicule, laugh, joke, or get angry, but quietly listen and speak slowly and calmly (in a low, even-toned voice) as most activities can be stopped with very little fuss
    - Provide a firm, polite, kind request to stop, and redirect with another activity, and determine the actual cause of his behavior
    - Provide guidelines of interventions for the partner of a person with Alzheimer's for when he behaves in a *sexually aggressive manner*:
        - Develop a crisis management plan with staff and family; plan for assistance in an emergency; never attempt to manage alone, and always have a phone handy
        - Avoid overreacting, especially forcefully, and avoid

Sexuality Concerns and Illness

anger and a moral attitude
- Move slowly, quietly, confidently, and place self between partner and the door, stand at a right angle; not directly in front of him or her
- Assess to determine whether the partner responds to verbal direction and, if able, attempt to de-escalate the situation
- Protect self before love, loyalty, or feelings of guilt

G. Potential Outcomes
- "Partner's feelings may not change towards the person they are caring for at all—they may find that they can connect with their partner through sex even if they are finding it difficult to communicate in other ways"[1(p2)]
- Some partners who are caregivers feel exhausted by their caring responsibilities and do not feel they have the energy to enjoy sex; this can be frustrating for the partner
- Some partners find that the intimate tasks they perform for a person with dementia puts them off being sexual with him (or her), which can make him feel that he has lost his dignity and affect how he feels about himself and his partner
- Many people find it hard to enjoy a sexual relationship if many other aspects of the relationship have changed and little else is shared, which can make it feel that sex has no

meaning. If lack of enjoyment is the case, it is important to give a person with dementia plenty of reassurance and affection in appropriate ways
- Some people feel that the dementia can make their partners clumsy or inconsiderate in bed. If so, the partner needs to be proactive and find new ways to be intimate together—whether or not this involves sex
- "Depending on how the dementia affects their relationship, some partners continue to sleep in the same bed as their partners while others choose to move to single beds or separate rooms. This can prove disconcerting or distressing for the person with dementia"[1(p3)]

Cancer and Sexuality

A. **Definition.** The presence of cancer and its associated treatments, with their emotionally and physically invasive effects on a person with cancer, frequently affect a person's perceptions of his or her sexuality, self-worth, and self-esteem.

B. **Signs and Symptoms**
- Side effects of cancer that directly or indirectly affect patient sexuality include pain, nausea and vomiting, anorexia, weight loss or weight gain, and osteoporosis; lowered self-esteem, unhappiness with body image, lymphadenopathy

post mastectomy, and depression; fear, anxiety, and grief; anemia; body hair loss, sleep disturbance, and fatigue, among others
- Patient may demonstrate embarrassment, hesitancy, or difficulty making statements about or asking questions of partner, family, and healthcare professionals about sexuality. It is especially difficult for patients who are gay, lesbian, bisexual, or transgender and have not previously shared this information; they have the added anxiety of the fear of prejudice
- Reduction in desire and libido, engorgement, arousal, and orgasm with cancer

C. Origins
- "Reduced desire and libido occur as a result of tiredness, stress, mood changes (such as anxiety), changes in contraception methods, feeling unhappy about your body; relationship problems, traumatic sexual experiences in the past, excessive drug or alcohol use, boredom with sexual routine."[3(p15)] If the patient is depressed, anxious, or afraid about cancer and treatments, it is usually difficult to become aroused
- In addressing patients, Macmillan Cancer Support states, "There are four main ways that cancer or its treatment can affect your sexuality. It can affect your:

- physical ability to give and receive sexual pleasure
- thoughts and feelings about your body (body image)
- emotions—such as fear, sadness, anger, and joy
- roles and relationships—if there's a problem in one of them, it may impact another"[3(p16)]
- The effects of cancer and its associated treatments on sexuality depend upon the cancer's location and stage and the type of treatment provided
- Macmillan Cancer Support identifies the following effects of cancer treatment on sexuality:
  - **Adverse effects of cancer surgery** on sexuality include nerve damage, sensory and vascular changes, scarring and disfigurement, vaginal and vulval changes (cervical and vulval cancers), mastectomy, the perceived loss of maleness in men (after an orchidectomy or prostatectomy) or femaleness in women (after a hysterectomy or oophorectomy)[3]
  - **Adverse effects of radiation therapy for cancer** on sexuality: hormonal changes; skin sensitivity and changes in elasticity especially of the groin, perineum, vulva, anal area; lymphedema; vaginal changes; and skin fragility. Pelvic floor irradiation may cause diarrhea, nausea, pain, and bleeding in women that are mostly temporary. Pregnancy is an extremely difficult issue to manage, especially if a female patient is already

impregnated. Radiation of the pelvic area may cause permanent hormonal changes in a woman that will induce a chemical menopause, resulting in hot flashes, dry vagina, and mood swings. Radiation adversely affects a man's erectile function due to scarring of the blood vessels, and consequently reduces blood supply to the penis[3]

- **Adverse effects of chemotherapy for cancer** on sexuality: peripheral neuropathy, mucosal inflammation of the vagina, vaginal dryness and candida: pubic and head hair loss, chemically-induced menopause, nausea, and vomiting; weakness, depression, tiredness, loss of libido; and weight loss/gain, vaginal atrophy, erectile dysfunction, reduced fertility, tiredness, and infertility[3]
- **Adverse effects of hormone therapy for cancer** on sexuality: anti-oestrogens can increase early menopausal symptoms, exacerbate vaginal dryness, and vaginal atrophy, reduce libido in women, and loss of fertility in women. Men experience loss of libido, loss of muscle strength, less semen, loss of fertility and diminished sexual feeling. Steroids increase blood glucose in men and women[3]

D. **Background**
- A survey of women who had breast cancer showed that a

third of all women, and half of those under age 55, have sex less often as a result of their cancer, and sexual problems are the most common long-term consequences of cancer, affecting around 35,000 people per year in the UK[3]
- Cancer-related fatigue is defined by the National Comprehensive Cancer Network as "A distressing, persistent, subjective sense of physical, emotional, and or cognitive tiredness or exhaustion related to cancer or cancer treatment that is not proportional to recent activity and interferes with usual functioning "to include sexuality and intimacy"[4(p2)]

E$_1$. Medical Interventions for Female Patient Sexuality Post Cancer Surgery (Macmillan Cancer Support, 2012)[3]
- Establish rapport with the patient, provide support, and encourage verbalization of sexual problems by patient with or without partner involvement
- Refer the patient to a sex therapist, psychologist, or advanced practice nurse if indicated
- Advise patient and partner against deep penetrative sex post-hysterectomy, as well as the potential for a *different-feeling* orgasm
- Share with the woman and partner that she will be infertile post-hysterectomy and discuss methods to preserve fertility potential

Sexuality Concerns and Illness

- Prescribe estrogen for chemical menopause symptoms
- Provide support and actively listen to the woman post-mastectomy since she will no longer experience sexual arousal via her breasts and the feelings associated with breast loss may equate to no longer feeling like a woman
- Prepare patient carefully and ensure that the patient is aware of the residual effects of abdominal-perineal resection, to include removal of the anus, rectum, and lower part of the colon and a stoma formed for the passage of feces. May include removal of the uterus, ovaries, and part of the vaginal wall. Encourage and provide open and frank dialogue to the patient about the life and sexual ramifications of a stoma and chemical menopause
- Acknowledge the additional difficulties of patients post-cancer surgery who are transgender and manage them appropriately (with psychologist and sex therapist input)

E_2. Therapeutic Interventions for Male Patients Post-Cancer Surgery

- Perform a Standard Sexual Assessment (Appendix C) and medical assessment, and obtain a sexual and medical history
- Establish rapport with patient, provide support, and encourage verbalization of sexual problems by patient with or without partner involvement

- Refer the patient to a sex therapist or sexologist, psychologist, dietician, social worker, home care nurse, physical therapist, and an advanced practice nurse where indicated
- Discuss with male patients that after a radical prostatectomy, men find it difficult to obtain and maintain an erection; no semen is produced, and any sperm produced will be reabsorbed rather than be ejaculated. Infertility will result
- Ensure that the patient is informed about sperm storage prior to surgery (if he desires future children)
- Inform the patient that during a cystectomy, a male patient will also have his prostate removed, which makes it impossible to have an erection; consequently, dry ejaculations will result
- Bladder resection is sometimes possible, or a stoma on the skin created for urinary drainage that will also affect sexuality
- Explain that an abdominal-peritoneal resection (AP) is performed for cancer of the rectum, in which the anus, rectum, and part of the lower end of the large bowel are removed. Ensure that the patient fully understands that anal sex will no longer be possible and a stoma necessary
- Inform the patient that removal of one or both testicles will result in a loss of libido, difficulty getting or maintaining an erection, and less intense orgasms. Prescribe hormone

Sexuality Concerns and Illness

  replacement when indicated
- Prepare the patient that surgery for cancer of the penis may involve partial or complete removal of his penis; this is usually devastating for a male patient to hear. Penile reconstruction is possible, and sexual arousal possible because of the sexual sensitivity of the scrotum, perineum, and testicles
- Acknowledge the additional difficulties of patients post-cancer surgery who are transgender and manage them appropriately, with psychologist or sexologist input

F. Supportive Interventions
- Review the Supportive Interventions Guide for Adults (Appendix H)
- Involve patient's partner when discussing sexual difficulties
- An experienced sexologist is advisable when teaching patients about new sexual positions and new sexual activities, one who is cognizant and respectful of the patient's values
- Ensure the pain is managed to an acceptable level of relief, adequate oral, intravenous, and supplemental fluids, and all medications administered (anti-emetics, usually prior to meals, chemotherapy medications on time/as ordered; administer analgesics on a regular schedule, and administer antibiotics on time as ordered)

- Careful attention to management of cancer symptoms will enhance sexuality potential
- Discuss the use of alternative therapy, such as acupuncture, and complementary therapies, such as music, relaxation techniques, and guided imagery to help alleviate pain
- Request the patient and partner arrange for sexual activities when patient is not fatigued, usually in the morning, and plan for naps
- If female patient is embarrassed about a mastectomy scar, encourage coverage with a bra or camisole; if a male patient is conscious of an abdominal scar, advise coverage with a T-shirt the first few times of sexual activity
- Monitor exercise regime and physical response to sexual activities to ensure patient does not get too tired
- Encourage patient to stop smoking and drinking alcohol, and provide intervention methods for both once patient in agreement
- Administer vaginal lubricants (water soluble) for female patient vaginal dryness

G. Potential Outcomes
- Some patients and their partners continue their sexual activities as previously; people who enjoyed a regular sexual life before cancer are usually more apt to do so after the cancer diagnosis

- Some patients and partners find that their previous thoughts/actions on sexuality change, and are replaced by ones of comfort, touch, intimacy, tenderness, love, and support
- Some patients and partners initially may lose their interest in sexuality but regain it after treatments stop and life is back to normal. However, sexual activities are usually not as active as previously
- Some patients and partners never resume their sexual activities after patient cancer; some are content with this arrangement, others are not

Diabetes Mellitus and Sexuality

A. **Definition.** "Diabetes is a complex group of diseases with a variety of causes. People with diabetes have high blood glucose, also called high blood sugar or hyperglycemia. Diabetes is a disorder of metabolism—the way the body uses digested food for energy. The digestive tract breaks down carbohydrates—sugars and starches found in many foods—into glucose, a form of sugar that enters the bloodstream. With the help of a hormone (insulin), cells throughout the body absorb glucose and use it for energy. Diabetes develops when the body doesn't make enough insulin or is not able to use the insulin effectively, or both"[5 (p1)]

B. Signs and Symptoms

- Early onset and increased severity of sexual problems, as well as problems with retrograde ejaculation and associated infertility, especially erectile problems in men
- Diminished sexual response and limited vaginal lubrication in women
- Uncomfortable and painful intercourse for women due to yeast and candida infections
- Urinary tract infections, urinary incontinence, and overactive bladder[6]

C. Origins

- Diabetes results in diabetic neuropathy, a condition that produces diminished peripheral feelings, pain, numbness, and tingling that are responsible for some of the sexual problems associated with diabetes
- Diabetes results in vascular changes that can cause numerous diseases. These include a blockage of the heart vessels that leads to hypertension, a condition that may result in a stroke or a heart attack, as well as blockage of leg vessels that may cause such diminished blood supply to the toes, feet, and legs, such that they may require amputation. The presence of these conditions impacts sexual interest, sexual arousal, and sexual performance[6]
- Retrograde ejaculation occurs with diabetes as a result of

Sexuality Concerns and Illness

   the loss of sphincter muscle tone of the bladder
- Erectile dysfunction (ED) is a common sexual problem in men with Type 2 diabetes
- Alcohol abuse, hypertension, smoking, cardiac problems, and other vascular problems often exacerbate the blood vessel and nerve damage begun by diabetes itself
- Poor control of diabetes may result in extremely labile (fluctuating) blood sugar levels; these in turn lead to hypoglycemia, especially during the night, and hyperglycemia, both of which may result in unconsciousness

D. Background
- Data from the largest study ever of quality of life in patients with diabetes revealed that one-third have ED that is related to health status perception. "In particular patients with ED showed higher levels of frustration and discouragement, and a lower acceptance of diabetes, which were, in turn, related to worse metabolic control and higher levels of depressive symptoms," De Bernardi et al. studied 615 male respondents and 34% reported frequent ED, 24% reported occasional ED, 42% were without erectile problems[7 (abstract)]
- "Of the patients reporting ED another important finding of this study is the dramatic increase in depression given by the concomitant presence of diabetes and ED; almost two-thirds of the patients reporting ED also had quality

of life values indicative of depressive symptoms. This prevalence is higher than reported in previous studies of diabetic adults"[7 (abstract)]

E. Therapeutic Interventions
- Perform a Standard Sexual Assessment (Appendix C) and medical assessment, and obtain a sexual and medical history
- Monitor all parameters of diabetes (especially blood sugars and A1c) to ensure disease is well-controlled because this will contribute to an overall improvement in patient sexuality
- Referral to an experienced sexologist is advisable when teaching patients about new sexual positions and new sexual activities; one who is cognizant of and respectful of the patient's values
- Prescribe Viagra, Cialis, or Levitra and caution patient about potential for low blood pressure if patient takes nitrates
- Encourage use of a different type of vibrator to increase arousal
- Prescribe water-based lubricants for vaginal dryness
- If retrograde ejaculation occurs, it sometimes responds to medications to improve bladder muscle sphincter control; if not successful, surgical intervention most often is

- Observe for depression, and if present, treat with antidepressants
- Discuss the potential for infertility and methods of sperm retrieval

F. Supportive Interventions
- Review the Supportive Interventions Guide for Adults (Appendix H)
- Maintain all the treatments and medications to halt the adverse actions of diabetes on sexuality
- Encourage an open dialogue between patient and partner about their sexuality, provide supportive educational materials for identified issues, and answer their questions
- Continue the dialogue with the patient and partner about use of a vibrator to stimulate arousal
- Support and encourage use of different positions for sexual intercourse to alleviate pain and reduce the potential for injury
- Discuss the use of water-based vaginal lubricants for vaginal dryness
- Teach about the risk factors associated with diabetes and their impact on blood vessels and all body systems, including smoking, obesity, hypertension, elevated cholesterol, and older than age 40; sedentary life, poor blood glucose control, fatigue, and hormonal deficiencies, all of which directly and indirectly affect sexuality

G. **Potential Outcomes**
- As control of diabetes is reached, the sexual problems experienced often improve
- Conversely, if control of diabetes is not reached, and risk factors not discontinued (especially smoking and high blood sugar levels), the sexual issues continue and worsen
- Associated depression about sexual issues, especially ED, increases and impacts other activities of daily living
- Complications associated with out-of-control diabetes, to include amputation, heart disease, and obesity, lead to a physically compromised patient, and sexual activities then may be beyond his or her reach

"Sex is more than an act of pleasure, it's the ability to be able to feel so close to a person, so connected, so comfortable it's almost breathtaking, to the point you feel you can't take it. And at this moment you're part of them."
— Sophia Loren

Multiple Sclerosis and Sexuality

A. **Definition.** Multiple Sclerosis (MS) is an immune-mediated process in which an abnormal response of the body's immune system is directed against the central nervous system, which comprises the brain, spinal cord, and optic nerve. The exact antigen or target that the immune cells are sensitized to attack remains unknown[8]

B. **Signs and Symptoms**
- Numbness of genitals, increased or decreased genital sensitivity, and decreased vaginal lubrication with associated vaginal dryness
- Difficult to achieve and/or maintain an erection, with ejaculation and orgasm problems
- Fatigue, muscle spasms, spasticity, and associated pain that makes sex painful and "positionally" difficult
- Loss of bladder and bowel control that is hard to ignore during sex
- Reduced self-esteem, concern, and sadness over changed body image
- Anger, stress, depression, and marital issues inhibit sexual activity
- Loss of sexual desire due to fatigue

C. **Origins**
- The secondary effects associated with MS contribute to sexual dysfunctions in both men and women. These side effects include fatigue, muscle spasticity, bowel and bladder problems, vaginal dryness, diminished blood supply, increased sensation, lowered self-esteem, and poor body image

D. Background
- MS is a condition that impacts people from an early age; initial symptoms may occur in a person in his or her early 20s, with a worsening of symptoms presenting in his or her 40s; consequently, the impact of sexual dysfunction on sexuality is experienced earlier than usual
- Although the actual incidence is difficult to obtain, it is estimated that between 2 to 2.5 million people worldwide have MS. It affects all ethnic groups, although people from some specific areas get the disease and others do not; it appears to be dependent on the distance from the equator. The farther people are from the equator and the more temperate the climate, the greater the prevalence. MS is unheard of in the Inuits, Yakutes, Hungarian Romany, Norwegian Lapps, Australian Aborigines, and New Zealanders[9]
- Many patients with MS want sexual relationships and to have children
- Two to three times more prevalent in women than men

E. Therapeutic Interventions
- Perform a Standard Sexual Assessment (Appendix C) and medical assessment, and obtain a sexual and medical history
- Maintain all current medications, especially those to

Sexuality Concerns and Illness

    control MS side effects
- Recommend use of genital vibrator to assist slow arousal, analgesics for increased genital sensitivity, and lubricants (water-soluble only) for vagina dryness
- ED is helped by use of a penile vacuum device, penile injection, suppositories, or penile implant, and/or oral Viagra, Levitra, or Cialis
- Oral medications for spasm control, together with physical therapy to enhance range of motion and promote muscle stretching. Avoid triggers of spasms such as tight clothing, incorrect positioning, and extremes in temperature and humidity
- Intermittent catheterization and medications such as imipramine for urinary leakage and incontinence and routine bowel evacuation methods for bowel control
- Encourage to explore on her own body—the feel, texture, and sensations—and find out what hurts, what does not, and share the results with her partner. Talk less about the disease process and hurt and more about sensuality and feelings
- Advise to remove sexual intercourse as her only sexual activity, and reduce performance fears
- Prescribe Sensate Focus, bibliotherapy, guided imagery, and visual erotica
- Discuss methods to increase intimacy and closeness with

partner, to include the use of touch, sensory stimulation, fantasy, different sexual activities, and added sexual techniques and different sexual positions
- Counseling, medications, and supportive therapy for marital, self-esteem, and body-image issues
- Refer to an experienced sex therapist when teaching patients about new sexual positions and new sexual activities; one considerate of and respectful of the patient's values

F. Supportive Interventions
- Review the Supportive Interventions Guide for Adults (Appendix H)
- Encourage patient to discuss her sexual concerns with her partner
- Discuss and demonstrate use of a vibrator and other *sex toys*, with careful attention paid to patient values
- Support the suggestions of the sex therapist following discussion of new sexual positions and techniques
- Demonstrate application and use of penile vacuum device; monitor self-administration of penile injections and use of the penile implant
- Discuss methods to control urinary and bowel incontinence
- Be involved in the routine nursing care of the patient's skin and prevention of contractures; provide supportive therapy and monitor for status of MS associated with sexual problems

- Encourage all prescribed interventions, with an emphasis on partner intimacy and discussion

G. **Potential Outcomes**
- The ability to have sexual intercourse and to reach orgasm may decrease as the symptoms of MS increase; however, these abilities are often replaced by increased intimacy and closeness with partner
- Sexual fulfillment may be achieved through sensual touch, sexual fantasy, sexual exploration, erotica, guided imagery, and other methods to increase intimacy
- Fatigue and pain may discourage attempts at sexual activities, but intimacy mostly prevails

"Sex is a wonderful function. You can't make it happen but you can teach people to let it happen."

— William Masters

Intellectual, Physical, and Developmental Disabilities and Sexuality

A. Definitions. Sexuality and its implications for the health and wellbeing of individuals who have either an intellectual, physical, or developmental disability

"An **intellectual disability** is characterized by significant limitations both in intellectual functioning (reasoning, learning, problem-solving) and in adaptive behavior which covers a range of everyday social and practical skills. This disability originates before age 18."[10(p1)] Examples include Down syndrome, autism, and Asperger's syndrome, among others.

A **physical disability** is a disability that affects a person's physical functioning, to include mobility and dexterity, or an impairment of breathing, vision, hearing, and/or speech a person is born with or acquires. Examples include spinal cord injury, cerebral palsy, hearing loss, amputation, spina bifida, cerebral vascular accidents, and congestive heart failure[11]

"A **developmental disability** is an umbrella term that includes intellectual disability but also includes other disabilities that are apparent during childhood. Developmental disabilities are severe chronic disabilities that can be cognitive or physical or both. These disabilities occur before age 22 and are likely to be lifelong."[10(p1)]

B$_1$. Signs and Symptoms
- People with an intellectual disability usually lack organized and accurate sexual information and understanding, which, together with a non-accepting society, leave them ill-prepared and confused, with feelings of low self-worth and self-confidence

- Instances of sexual abuse by able-bodied persons may occur, often with weak, implausible justifications for the abuse by the perpetrator such as "She enjoyed it," "I am doing her a favor," or "She knew what she was doing."
- Frequently the sexual abuse is first noticed by the presence of STIs in both males and females or pregnancy in a woman. Often the person with an intellectual disability may have no awareness of the STI and sometimes not even the pregnancy
- Complaints by persons (especially with an intellectual disability) of being victims of stigmatization, with its associated signs and symptoms that include clinical depression, labile emotions, inability to socialize, and diminished self-worth and self-esteem. Also, complaints of being dehumanized as an object of fear and ridicule with the internalization of inaccurate depictions of them such as being stupid, comical, laughable, or even ugly[10]
- Most people get their sex education from parents, school, their peers, and the media; this is not the case for intellectually disabled people. Most often, sex education, when it is provided, is given by parents who are often overworked, anxious, and caring, but often lack the knowledge and teaching ability, and the information provided may be inaccurate or incomplete

B$_2$. Signs and Symptoms

- The most frequent complaints of men with a physical

disability are erectile dysfunction and ejaculation issues (which depend upon the severity and location of the physical injury), followed by infertility concerns. Women with a physical disability complain mostly about lack of sexual arousal, lack of lubrication, and loss of tactile sensation
- Men and women with a spinal cord injury both have episodes of spasticity during sex
- Men and women with a spinal cord injury have both sexual thoughts, desires, and fantasies, but their physical disability interferes with their ability to achieve their sexual thoughts
- Some have mobility difficulties that result in an inability to attain certain sexual positions, some are unable to thrust effectively, and some are unable to contract certain muscles
- Many young men and women with a spinal cord injury want to have children and are interested in sex
- Men usually have more sexual issues than women after an injury, not only because of their anatomical differences to women, but also the perceived threat to their manhood, which may become overwhelming for them
- Persons with a physical disability may express beliefs that they feel sexually unattractive, are unable to live up to societal expectations of what is attractive, and are less worthy of sexual partners or sexual relationships than persons without a disability[11]

B₃. Signs and Symptoms

- As previously stated, developmental disability is an umbrella term that includes not only intellectual disability and physical disability, but also includes other disabilities that become apparent during childhood
- The same signs and symptoms described previously for intellectual and physical disabilities are also demonstrated by persons with a developmental disability. However, their sexual concerns are often magnified as they have the added challenges of having both intellectual and physical disabilities and having to contend with their signs and symptoms

C. Origins

- "There are a number of causes. Our understanding of the causes of intellectual disability focuses on the types of risk factors (biomedical, social, behavioral, and educational) and the timing of exposure (prenatal, perinatal, and postnatal) to those factors."[10 (p1)]
- Anecdotally, it is suggested that there are about 200 causes of intellectual disabilities, a few of which are maternal infection, behavior (fetal alcoholism, effects of smoking), malnutrition, disease, environmental; premature infant, low infant birth weight, traumatic delivery, among many others

D. Background

- People with an intellectual disability are denied their sexuality by the stigma assigned by society, imposed economic constraints, absence of standard physical appearance, and society's fear of disabled persons having children who are also disabled and unable to take care of themselves[12]
- The accurate number of people who are disabled worldwide is impossible to determine, although it has been suggested that 50% of disabled people do not have any form of sex life at all[9]
- Some able-bodied people are of the opinion that people with an intellectual disability have no sexual rights at all, they de-sexualize them, and they see them as completely asexual. They see them as without sensual, intimacy, affection, bonding, or parenting needs
- When people with a disability do exhibit any sexual behaviors, some call them oversexed and treat them negatively; some even say, "They don't need sex education; they need to be castrated or sterilized."
- "Sexuality is often equated just with sex. Actually it is much broader and also encompasses gender identity and roles, sexual orientation, eroticism, pleasure, intimacy and reproduction. Sexuality is experienced and expressed in thoughts, fantasies, desires, beliefs, attitudes, values,

Sexuality Concerns and Illness

behaviors, practices, roles, and relationships. It is influenced by psychological, economic, political, social, and biological factors. Sexuality is a natural and healthy aspect of living, and it is part of who we are. Women with disabilities are rarely seen as sexual beings, however. This leads to a range of myths and misconceptions around their sexuality...such as:[13]

- "Women with disabilities do not need sex
- Women with disabilities are not sexually attractive
- Women with disabilities are 'oversexed'
- Women with disabilities have more important needs than sex
- Girls living with disabilities do not need sexuality education
- Women who live with disabilities cannot have 'real' sex
- Sex must be spontaneous
- Women with disabilities should not have children" [13 (p1)]
- Other myths and misconceptions are that people with an intellectual disability are either not interested in sex, not capable, or are overly interested in sex and out of control with their sexual activities
- Some able-bodied people, upon learning that a person has a disability, are not interested in forming intimate or even friendly relationships with that person. They fear the disabled person being dependent on them, having to

333

care physically for the person and financially support him or her, or losing their current social standing by having a close relationship with a disabled person[12]
- Men who have a disability are placed into a secondary slot in life, with a lesser social standing, community position, and economic standing. In a society where beauty is overvalued, those who are beautiful are always regarded more highly, especially when compared to the woman who is disabled[12]

E. Therapeutic Interventions
- Perform a Standard Sexual Assessment (Appendix C) and medical assessment, and obtain a sexual and medical history
- Perform a physical and sexual assessment and obtain a sexual and medical history
- Reassure the person who has a spinal cord injury, or another physical injury, that sexual satisfaction is still attainable, but the sexual approaches, positions, activities, etc. will change
- Advise that direct and honest communication between the patient and his partner is paramount
- Referral to an experienced sex therapist is advisable when teaching patients about new sexual positions and new sexual activities; one who is considerate and respectful of

the patient's values
- Determine whether patient is a candidate for Viagra, Cialis, or Levitra for erectile dysfunction, and describe the drug's efficacy and efficiency, as well as the potential for autonomic dysreflexia during sexual activity and nitrate use
- Determine whether the male patient is a potential candidate for vacuum therapy, penile injections, vibratory stimulation, or a penile implant for ED, and evaluate potential for treatment for infertility if needed
- Counsel the parents of a child with an intellectual disability to reinforce protection methods that apply to potential sexual abuse of their child, and ensure that the sexual education for the child is appropriate and accurate
- Provide information to the parents or caregivers of a child with an intellectual disability to his or her level of comprehension about opposite sex friendships and relationships, sex education, birth control, STIs, AIDs, and a safe community and work environment

F_1. Supportive Interventions
- Review the Supportive Interventions Guides for Children and Adults (Appendices G and H)
- Develop policies about "The right to privacy and dignity, the right to accessible information and guidance, the right to counselling as appropriate, the right to their body integrity

and how this can be protected, in accordance with their ability to protect themselves"[12]
- Always address persons with an intellectual disability in an age-appropriate, respectful, non-condescending manner, and provide time for them to respond to questions, observations, etc.
- Always dress the person who is disabled in age-appropriate and occasion-appropriate clothes; if an adult, avoid the use of bows in her hair, pigtails, ankle socks, etc. Reinforce her attractiveness without being overly *effuse* and unrealistic
- Teach the patient ways to protect self
- Dispel the myths listed above and teach self and others:[13(p1-3)]
  - Not to treat people (especially women) with a disability as though they are children or as being genderless; all humans are sexual beings throughout all their lives
  - That sexual attraction is a physical and emotional connection between two people with which the standards imposed by society have no connections or controls whatsoever
  - That the perception that intellectually disabled girls and women are *oversexed* is more about a person's lack of education about what is sexually appropriate or inappropriate than a biological condition
  - Sexual desires are not secondary to other physical and emotional needs for disabled persons and should not be treated as such

Sexuality Concerns and Illness

- Regardless of age, religion, culture, with or without a disability, we all need sex education. People with a disability may or may not need more; however, what they receive may need to be presented in a different format to facilitate comprehension and understanding
- Sex is for everyone, regardless of presence or absence of a disability
- Even though preparations often need to be completed prior to sex for a disabled person, this is actually the case for all of us; we all prepare in some way or another; it is rarely spontaneous. The difference is that the preparations are somewhat different and may involve equipment, devices, appliances, lubricants, etc.
- People with a disability are no more prone to have a child who is disabled than a person without a disability; very few disabilities are hereditary[13]
- Teach the person with an intellectual disability and others about health-related issues, appropriate sexual behavior, reproduction and pregnancy, and sexuality rights[14]
- Provide education and supportive literature about sexuality and being disabled to children, parents, teachers, among others at their appropriate reading level and level of comprehension
- Educate about sex and sexuality, with special attention paid to aspects that impact persons with a specific

disability. For example, persons with spina bifida are allergic to latex, so latex condoms and dental dams are to be avoided; persons in a wheelchair for great lengths of time may be more prone to a thrombus and oral contraception should be avoided[13(p1-3)]

- "Because people who are disabled are often vulnerable to sexual abuse, prevention information should be readily available. Allowing myth to take over reason could also mean unnecessary exposure to sexually transmitted diseases, including the fatal consequences of contracting acquired immunodeficiency syndrome (AIDS)."[14(p1)]

F_2. Supportive Interventions

- Review the Supportive Interventions Guide for Adults (Appendix H)
- Teach that communication, experimentation, and exploration between the two partners are the cornerstones to retention of an active sexual life for a person with an acquired disability, and that having a disability does not mean that sexuality is a thing of the past. It may be less enjoyable or more enjoyable; however, it will be different
- Ensure that the person with a disability and partner receive information on family planning, contraceptive counseling and service, sex therapy service by a qualified person, and

advice about the prevention and detection of sexual abuse
- Reinforce information about medications prescribed and over-the-counter drugs patient uses
- Demonstrate use of sex devices to treat ED in men such as penile vacuum pumps, manual stimulation pumps, memory foam position wedges, sex toys, vibrators, or devices such as the Intimate Rider Sex chair to optimize penile thrusting
- Discuss the use of Viagra, Cialis, and Levitra and their potential for successful treatment of ED in men. So far not helpful in women
- Teach patient how to manage bowel and bladder control, and management of catheter or intermittent catheterization, especially before and during sexual activity
- Reinforce information about the potential with Viagra, etc., for autonomic dysreflexia and potential for severe hypotension to occur during sexual activity and warn of its associated dangers with nitrates

G. Potential Outcomes
- Many men and women with an acquired physical disability are able to resume an active and satisfactory sex life; however, for some, their perceptions of being unattractive, clumsy, and worthless may impede their actual resumption of sexual activities
- Sexual activities are different for the person who is recently

- physically disabled; however, they can be rewarding if intimacy, touch, affection, tenderness, experimentation, massage, and communication are active factors in their relationship
- Physical and emotional aspects of sexuality can be maintained, but some people with a physical disability may become too fatigued, disillusioned, or anxious, and dejected with the sexual process, and may just give up their efforts. This may lead to partner discontent and relationship issues
- A male with a spinal cord injury who desires to be a father may do so by retrieval and insemination of sperm into the woman's uterus
- Males and females with an intellectual disability still face the potential for being sexually abused, of contracting STIs and the female becoming pregnant or the male impregnating a female
- Unethical people may insist on non-consensual birth control, chemical castration, or sterilization for the person who is intellectually disabled

Disrespect, verbal abuse, physical abuse, ridicule, and other adverse behaviors toward persons with a disability continue today; however, the rights of persons with a disability have been brought to the public platform, certainly in the Western world, and increased awareness has taken place.

Older Individuals and Sexuality

Being older (let us say over the age of 65) does not necessarily mean that men and women have absolutely no interest in sex; quite the contrary. Too often, the automatic assumptions of younger people, for example an HCP in her middle 30s, are that the silver-haired man sitting down in front of her with cane in his hand never thinks about sex, does not want sex, and certainly never has sex. Not so. He may walk slowly and rise a little hesitantly from a chair, but that does not mean he is not interested in sex, and certainly does not mean he does not want to or does not actually participate. Some older persons may not be interested in sexual activities for many reasons, but for a great number of individuals, their sexuality remains, and they want it to remain a great part of their lives.

The prevailing assumption is that because older men and women have fewer male and female sex hormones, they are automatically placed into the menopausal group, which translated, means they cannot, and do not, want to do anything sexual, and never consider participating in sexual activities. Obviously, many older individuals have problems associated with older age; less agility and dexterity, bodily fatigue, limb weakness, an ostomy, pain, visual and auditory changes, being without a current partner, pain, or bone and limb issues, among others, that can all result in diminished sexual activities. Some men may not attain or maintain a stiff erection, and some women may have less vaginal lubrication than they would like. However, do not mistake a person of an older age with an illness or who is less than able-bodied with being a person who is incapable of having sexual activities that result in sexual pleasure for both partners.

There are also many benefits to getting older. Freedom from fears of pregnancy, freedom from care of their young children with their squabbles, interruptions, and distractions, and associated worries; freedom from financial worries, from employment challenges, from the need to get ahead professionally; freedom from disastrous love affairs, with their tears and jealousy; freedom from in-laws; the list is virtually endless. Things also seem better about one's personal self: increased self-confidence, higher self-esteem, fewer worries (especially what others think about you), love of family, partner, children, and grandchildren.

"We have good news for the physically limited and sexually dysfunctional: Full sexual functionality is not necessary for optimal sexuality. There is bad news for the physically healthy: Full sexual functionality is not sufficient for wonderful sex."

— Kleinplatz, Maynard, Paradis, Campbell, Dalgeish, Segovia et al.

Sexuality Concerns and Illness

This section does not repeat discussion of sexual problems and interventions as they are described in previous sections (primarily Chapter 8: Sexual Disorders), but addresses the changes associated with older age that impact sexual activities and result in what are labeled as sexual problems. Gender, either male or female, is used interchangeably within the text below as most suggestions can apply to both men and women. Where that is not the case, the other gender is specified, together with specific directions for interventions.

To facilitate effective therapeutic and supportive interventions that address an older person's sexual needs, the HCP is advised to:

- Follow all the guidelines for a sexual interview, or therapeutic or supportive interventions
- Evaluate his or her own perceptions and opinions about the elderly and ensure that any negative perceptions or opinions are eliminated or at least controlled during her time with the older patient. Of particular concern is an individual who is repulsed by the thought of older people participating in sexual activities; in this case, request reassignment
- Obtain the patient's awareness of contributing factors that may impact his sexuality, and determine what connections there are between his identified contributing factors and his current

343

sexuality issues
- Discuss his current medications for their effects on his sexuality
- Ensure that he and his partner are both aware of the symptoms of menopause in women and andropause in men. Menopause includes night sweats, absence of periods, irritability, headaches, hot flashes, labile emotions, and irritability in his female partner. Andropause or ADAM (androgen decline in aging male) is less dramatic and acute in onset and presents with depression, fatigue, tiredness, weakness
- Avoid downplay of his recent disappointing sexual activities, and encourage discussion of his solutions to the factors that contribute to that disappointment
- Advise that he discard the sexual scripts of his youth, and discuss elimination of the heterosexual script that designates sexual intercourse as the *Holy Grail* of sexual activities; it is just one of many. Encourage experimentation and creativity, and developing a new sexual script for himself
- Determine whether he has an intimate relationship with his partner. Promote emotional and physical intimacy as the staunch and steady companion of sexual activities in older people, without which attempts at a successful sexual relationship may fail
- Intimacy is perceived and described differently when people are asked. Some intimate acts include touching, smiling, sharing, loving, tenderness, unity/oneness, connecting, liking,

Sexuality Concerns and Illness

familiarity, comfortable and comforting, calmness and calming, appreciation, closeness, and friendship
- Advise him to work with his partner to *white flag* old battles, minimize small squabbles, and forgive any pettiness of years ago; doing so will reduce old baggage and old hurts that adversely affect intimacy and sexuality
- If there is an uncomfortably greater age difference between the man and his partner, male or female, advise him to discuss this openly with his partner so that both have the opportunity to share opinions. If they are in disagreement, or one wants secrecy, or one is fearful of societal opinion, or feels it is not worth the risk, best to consider an end to the relationship
- Remind that men and women have spent a great deal of time throughout their lifetimes in preparation for most of their sexual encounters (time spent to arrange a specific time, date, place, bathed, hair styled, attire, shoes, provocative (or just *nice*) underwear, perfume, travel to and from, etc.), and it is no different because the person is older. Advise to arrange for sexual activities in the early afternoon (if possible), when both not tired, having taken pain medications if needed. Ensure the room (any room, not just the bedroom) is not too warm or too cold, be sure to have pillows, a cover, a chair, sex gel and oil, a towel, sex toys and equipment (a vibrator, a dildo, a sex wedge, a sex swing, vacuum device, elastic bands, etc.)
- Be prepared, anticipate *operational problems,* but enjoy the

adventure
- Remind him to wear a condom or his female partner a dental dam even though they may be out of practice in application. Neither person is immune to acquiring an STI, passing an STI to his male or female partner, or a man to impregnating his female partner
- Caution that a full bladder that leaks may prove to be a damper on sex, so empty his bladder, or if catheterized, tape it down out of the way
- Remind the patient that the use of fantasy and erotica in its many forms is encouraged, either alone or with his partner—sensual and sexual books, romance books, movies, the Internet, paintings, magazines, among others
- If one or both partners have an illness, pain, muscle spasms, dexterity issues, or a disability that impedes sexual activities, advise the man and his partner to discuss and work through each obstacle, and experiment with positions, pillows, lubricants, massage, sex toys, sex devices, and wise use of pain medications
- Convey that the missionary style for intercourse may be painful and energetic, so modify his position and that of his partner that accommodates; do not hyperextend limbs, prevent spasms, and relieve pain. Obtain diagrams of positions and sexual activities that help reduce pain according to the disease from sex and disability organizations on the Internet, and modify your usual positions. For example, fellatio (oral sex) is much easier for a woman with an injured, painful back to perform on her male

Sexuality Concerns and Illness

partner than missionary style intercourse and cunnilingus (oral sex) for a man with an injured back to perform on his female partner.
- Anal sex may also benefit the situation
- Ensure male patient that oral sex is less stressful, and that a person's mouth contains more bacteria than the tip of a man's penis. Discussions about oral sex or anal sex and the female or male partner and their values and preferences are to be considered before attempted

"I am not saying everybody is involved with oral sex, but… the one thing I can say with assurance to you is that there is nothing abnormal about it."

— Dr. Ruth

- Advise to be totally engaged in sex and willing; if not, do not continue just for the sake of it; his body will eventually betray him and his partner will be aware
- Convey that it is not an increased frequency of the sexual activities that is sought, but the quality that he and his partner enjoy
- Request him to ask his partner to guide his or her hand gently to show what hurts, what does not, and what helps. Continue to show and tell each other until both are satisfied they are in

agreement and understand

- Tell him not to wait for an erection as it is not essential; however, if desire for sexual activities is present, then proceed. Partner may use warm sex oil to fondle softly and stroke gently if his penis is flaccid. If no success, the stop-start technique that is used for premature ejaculation can also be effective to tease the man and increase his arousal. Masturbation may complete arousal and erection. If not, his flaccid penis can be *stuffed* into his partner's vagina, or placed against his partner's anus. Both may increase arousal and partial or full erection
- Ask him to document their activities and the outcomes to evaluate success
- Convey your positive attitude toward sex in older people, and let your enthusiasm be infectious; bolster him and his partner with the knowledge and support they need
- Encourage the use of humor, laughter, and keeping conversations lighthearted during these experiments with positions and change in usual sexual practices; it will be fun and well worth the effort

Individuals in Their End-of-Life Illness and Sexuality

A. **Definition.** An end-of-life illness is the time when a person is in the terminal period of his or her life. This period may be experienced at home, in a hospice, a hospital, or an extended care facility setting. The person may be aware death is imminent, and he or she remains fully cognizant of feelings of love, intimacy, and affection.

B. **Signs and Symptoms**
- The European Association for Palliative Care (2004), in its assessment of sexuality of patients in palliative care, states that several themes emerged. One theme was that emotional connection to others was an integral component of sexuality, taking precedence over physical expressions. Sexuality continues to be important at the end of life"[15(abstract)]
- During this time, their final opportunity, people have a strong desire to express verbally their feelings of love and affection for the important people in their lives. Many times, they will physically express those feelings through touch, an embrace, a kiss, a look, holding hands, and patting

C. **Origins**
- Fatigue often precludes more strenuous sexual activities than those mentioned above. Cancer-related fatigue is defined by the National Comprehensive Cancer Network (in Keeney and Head)[16] as being a distressing, persistent, subjective sense of physical, emotional, and/or cognitive tiredness or exhaustion related to cancer or cancer treatment that is not proportional to recent activity and interferes

with usual functioning, to include sexuality and intimacy
- Severe anorexia and anemia also contribute to excessive fatigue and lack of demonstrated sexuality during a person's end-of-life-illness; similarly, nausea and vomiting inhibit most patient activities, to include their sexuality
- While they want to express their emotional feelings to those they love, some patients are embarrassed and unable to find and speak the right words
- Patients do not feel the surroundings are conducive; too stark, clinical, depressing, noisy, with too many people around

D. Background
- "Lack of privacy, shared rooms, staff intrusion and single beds were considered barriers to expressing sexuality in the hospital and hospice settings. Home care nurses and physicians were seen as the appropriate caregivers to address this issue. Subjects unanimously mentioned that a holistic approach to palliative care would include opportunities to discuss the impact of their illness on their sexuality"[15(abstract)]

E. Therapeutic Interventions
- Perform a Standard Sexual Assessment (Appendix C) and medical assessment, and obtain a sexual and medical history

Sexuality Concerns and Illness

- Work to rectify the lack of privacy for patients in healthcare facilities and staff intrusion into patient visits with loved ones through careful, detailed planning of facilities and staffing levels with administrative staff
- Involve experienced and empathetic nurses, a social worker, and a sex therapist to facilitate open discussion and recognition within the facility of the sexuality needs of patients at the end of their lives and promote a sex-positive environment
- Prescribe adequate pain control
- Provide lubricants and other support materials as needed

F. Supportive Interventions
- Review the Supportive Interventions Guide for Adults (Appendix H)
- Facilitate the sexual needs of the patient by meeting the physical, intellectual, and comfort needs. Ensure he or she is free of pain, is not too hot or too cold, positioned how wants to be, and comfortable and close to loved ones
- Severe anorexia contributes to excessive fatigue, so support dietary plan to include small meals (without drinks at the same time); provide nutrient-rich supplements and appetite stimulants, steroids to reduce the distress that surrounds anorexia,[16] and administer anti-emetics
- Prevent too much noise, too many people around, too many

interruptions, too many procedures, too many questions
- Help to get the patient home, if possible, to where the patient is able to express and demonstrate his or her feelings about sexuality comfortably

G. Potential Outcomes
- Patient is able to express his or her love, affection, and sexuality before he or she dies
- Patient is unable to express his or her love, affection, and sexuality before he or she dies

Points for Discussion:

Ask yourself : How comfortable am I with expressions of their sexuality by patients who have an end-of-life illness?

Ask yourself: How do I manage the observable discomfort of the patient's adult children that sometimes occurs? Is my approach effective and supportive?

CHAPTER 10
HIGH SEXUAL DESIRE DISORDERS AND SEXUAL COMPULSIVITY IN MEN AND WOMEN, AND THE LEARNED BEHAVIORS THAT CONTRIBUTE TO THEIR SEXUALLY COMPULSIVE ACTIONS

"...sex permeates all his thoughts and feelings, allowing no other aims in life, tumultuously, and in a rut-like fashion demanding gratification without granting the possibility of moral and righteous counter presentations, and resolving itself into an impulsive, insatiable succession of sexual employments."

— Krafft Von Ebing, Victorian Psychiatrist

1. High Sexual Desire Disorders and Sexual Compulsivity Disorders in Men

A. **Definition.** Kafka[1] provided three criteria for compulsive sexuality, a) recurrent, intense, sexually arousing fantasies, sexual urges, or behavior involving aspects of sexual expression that increase in frequency or intensity so as to interfere significantly with the expression for reciprocal, affectionate activity, b) these fantasies, urges, or behaviors cause significant distress or impairment socially or occupationally, and c) they do not occur during an episode of another DSM-IV Axis 1 condition, substance abuse, or other medical condition provided for compulsive sexuality.

B. **Signs and Symptoms**
   - Unwanted sexual desire, thoughts, impulses, and sexual activities, including sexual behaviors that are normative expressions of sexual desire and socially accepted but may become intrusive and excessive, to the exclusion of all other activities
   - Sexually compulsive behavior does not usually bring pleasure, just anxiety
   - Sexual activities include excessive sexual intercourse with multiple anonymous partners and one night stands; obsessive/excessive relationships; Internet pornography dependence; dependence on anonymous sexual outlets such as chat rooms, phone sex, use of prostitutes, excessive masturbation, excessive fantasy, and other

sexual compulsions[2]
- The more the man tries to stop, the worse he feels (anxiety, depression, and guilt); the worse he feels, the more he acts out sexually
- All activities are without emotional bonding or complete sexual satisfaction, and they are associated with guilt and shame
- Men are more aggressive and more diverse in their sexual activities than women

C. Origins
- Some consider this condition to be either an addiction, an obsessive-compulsive disorder, an impulse control disorder, and/or a high sexual desire
- Great controversy exists over the addiction label; many feel it is a contrived label for which there is no sound empirical evidence nor established criteria; it is not mentioned as a disorder in the recently published DSM-5
- Kafka[1] proposes that sexual addiction is an actual psychopathology associated with a loss of control over sexual behaviors as a response to negative emotions or life stressors
- The sexual addict was emotionally or sexually abused as a child with associated inadequate coping mechanisms, such as guilt, shame, and low self-esteem and worth

- The person has difficulty establishing emotional intimacy
- The sexual activity is associated with attempts to relieve anxiety and personal distress
- Environmental, hereditary aspects, and life's events may all be involved

D. Background
- These sexual activities are socially accepted, and they are not against the law; however, their excessive sexual activity, frequency, and intensity adversely impact activities of daily living for the man and ruin lives and relationships
- Men become skilled liars, planners, and schemers as they meticulously execute their plans
- High sexual desire, sexual activity, and compulsive sexual behaviors are more prevalent among men than women
- The excessive sexual behavior is associated with high risk behaviors such as alcohol, drug abuse, and unprotected sex
- Accurate prevalence is unknown since many men do not seek help, and those who do are usually forced by the legal system

E. Therapeutic Interventions
- Perform a Standard Sexual Assessment (Appendix C) and medical assessment, and obtain sexual and medical histories

- Psychotherapy, CBT, and self-help groups such as Twelve-Step programs (if the mental health professional advocates the addiction model)
- Prescribe pharmacotherapy with SSRIs such as sertraline, fluoxetine, fluvoxamine, and paroxetine to inhibit serotonin reuptake; tricyclic antidepressants such as imipramine and desipramine to inhibit serotonin reuptake; lithium to enhance serotonin function; and medroxyprogesterone to inhibit testosterone[2]

F. Supportive Interventions
- Review the Supportive Interventions Guide for Adults (Appendix H)
- Teach about the risks associated with a man's behavior. STIs from excessive visits to prostitutes; physical and emotional harm from excessive sexual activities; job, income and financial security loss; and isolation and withdrawal from partner, children, family, and friends
- Observe and question for signs of adverse effects of medications
- Obtain social service support for financial and family issues
- Implement couple therapy to assist with relationship and anxiety issues
- Implement supportive aspects of CBT

G. Potential Outcomes

- Constant feelings of diminished self-worth, guilt, anxiety, distress, depression, and despair may continue unless treated
- Incremental activities needed to meet escalating sexual desire and needs that lead to increased risk and harm to self and to others
- The need to stop is not as strong as the man's desire for the behavior to continue and escalate, and efforts to stop his behavior alone are not usually successful
- Sometimes symptoms can be treated successfully with counseling therapy and medication, but only if the treatment is strictly adhered to and continued

2. High Sexual Desire Disorders and Sexual Compulsivity in Women

A. Definition. The woman is totally obsessed with sexual thoughts and sexual activities to the exclusion of almost everything else. Her sexual activities are usually socially acceptable but intrusive and excessive, and if untreated, usually result in emotional, psychological, and physical distress

B. Signs and Symptoms

- Unwanted sexual desire, thoughts, impulses, and sexual

activities to include sexual behaviors that are normative expressions of sexual desire and socially accepted, but become intrusive and excessive to the exclusion of all other activities
- All sexual activities are without emotional bonding or sexual satisfaction, but with guilt, shame, and a marked impairment of daily activities

C. Origins
- Some psychologists and sexologists consider this condition to be either an addiction, an obsessive-compulsive disorder, an impulse control disorder, or hyper-sexuality. There is great controversy about the addiction label; many feel it is a contrived label for which there is no sound empirical evidence
- Paternal incest is identified as a potential origin as use of her body is the only way the woman learned she could get affection and attention from her father, and she then gravitates to other men
- May be associated with the origins of compulsive shopping, gambling, or exercise
- Environment, heredity, and life's events may all be involved

D. Background
- Previously known as nymphomania and considered to be a

mental health problem
- Less prevalent and mostly less intense in women than men
- Prevalence is unknown as many women never seek help and only then when forced by the legal system

E. Therapeutic Interventions
- Perform a Standard Sexual Assessment (Appendix C) and medical assessment, and obtain sexual and medical histories
- Psychotherapy, cognitive behavioral therapy (CBT), behavioral therapy, and self-help groups such as Twelve-Step programs (if the mental health professional advocates the addiction model)
- Prescribe pharmacotherapy with SSRIs such as sertraline, fluoxetine, fluvoxamine, paroxetine to inhibit serotonin reuptake; tricyclic antidepressants such as imipramine and desipramine to inhibit serotonin reuptake; lithium to enhance serotonin function; and medroxytestosterone to inhibit testosterone[16(p2)]

F. Supportive Interventions
- Review the Supportive Interventions Guide for Adults (Appendix H)
- Teach about the risks associated with the woman's behavior—STIs, unwanted pregnancy, physical and

emotional harm, loss of income, prostitution, and loss of friends/family support
- Administer and monitor medications
- Implement supportive aspects of CBT

G. Potential Outcomes
- Low self-esteem and poor self-worth; guilt, anxiety, distress, and incapacitating hopelessness and despair may continue if risky behaviors do not stop
- Increased activity needed to meet sexual needs that leads to increased risk and possible harm
- The need to stop is not as strong as her desire for the behavior to continue/escalate; efforts to stop her behavior without professional help are not usually successful
- Sometimes symptoms can be successfully treated with therapy and medications if both continued, and with family and social support

SECTION 6

DSM-5 IDENTIFIED PARAPHILIAS AND PARAPHILIC DISORDERS, DSM-5 SPECIFIED AND UNSPECIFIED PARAPHILIC DISORDERS AND OTHER PARAPHILIC DISORDERS

CHAPTER 11

A GENERAL OVERVIEW OF PARAPHILIAS AND PARAPHILIC DISORDERS. EIGHT DSM-5 SELECTED PARAPHILIAS AND PARAPHILIC DISORDERS, DSM-5 SPECIFIED AND UNSPECIFIED PARAPHILIAS AND PARAPHILIC DISORDERS, AND EXAMPLES OF NON-DSM-5 PARAPHILIC DISORDERS

"After the terror and fear of what I had done had left, which took about a month or two, I started it all over again. From then on it was a craving, a hunger.

"I don't know how to describe it, a compulsion, and I just kept doing it and doing it, whenever the opportunity presented itself."

— Jeffrey Dahmer

About every 10-15 years since 1952, American psychiatrists have written a book about medical conditions within the general public that they consider to be mental disorders. Written specifically for psychiatrists and other HCPs, this publication commands great respect and is used as a guide for many healthcare decisions about mental health that are made. Descriptions and management of the paraphilias are included, and the most recent edition, DSM-5 (*The Diagnostic and Statistical Manual of Psychiatric Disorders*, fifth edition) was published in May, 2013.

1. Sexual Paraphilias and Sexual Paraphilic Disorders: A General Overview

A. Definitions.

A_1. **Paraphilias** are defined as[1] recurrent, intense sexually arousing fantasies, sexual urges, or behaviors generally involving 1) non-human objects, 2) suffering humiliation of oneself or one's partner, or 3) children or other non-consenting persons that occur over a period of at least six months.

A_2. **Paraphilic disorders**[2] require that people with a paraphilia also feel "…personal distress about their interest, not merely distress resulting from society's disapproval; or have a sexual desire or behavior that involves another person's psychological distress, injury, or death, or a desire for sexual behaviors involving unwilling persons or persons unable to give legal consent."[p1]

Brannon[3] and associates condensed the above definitions and stated them more simply:

A. Definitions

A **Paraphilia** is any intense and persistent sexual interest other than sexual interest in genital stimulation or preparatory fondling with phenotypically normal, physically mature consenting human partners.[3]

A **Paraphilic disorder** is a paraphilia that causes distress or impairment to the individual or its satisfaction entails physical harm (or the risk of such harm) to others.[3]

B. Signs and Symptoms

- People, mostly males, with these conditions experience sexual arousal in response to stimulation from a specific object or sexual behavior and ritual that is not considered to be conventional sexual behavior, is not socially accepted, and is usually unlawful
- Personal distress occurs with many paraphilic disorders, especially the so-called hands-on paraphilic disorders (e.g., pedophilia) and somewhat less with the hands-off paraphilic disorders (fetishism, transvestic fetishism)
- "Although several of these disorders can be associated with

aggression or harm, others are neither inherently violent nor aggressive (e.g., fetishism, transvestic fetishism); and most do not invade another's personal space"[4 (p1)]
- The person with a paraphilia demonstrates very little interest in any aspects of his other life outside his life-consuming paraphilia activities, and he is often guilt-ridden, withdrawn, introverted, and unsociable
- He creates a sexual fantasy world for himself to substitute for real intimacy that he is usually not able to attain in real life
- The person with a paraphilia has irrational and distorted thoughts and ideas, and is often socially inept
- It is estimated that the majority of people with a paraphilia or a paraphilia-related disorder present with depression as a result of their condition and its impact on their lives
- Some men may suffer from relationship issues, low self-esteem, chronic under-employment, occupational difficulties, financial issues, guilt, and shame
- A social stigma is attached to the assignment of a mental disorder label that often results in despair and loneliness for many of these individuals
- Each paraphilia or paraphilic behavior is extremely complex and varies in its specific presentation (greater detail follows of specific paraphilias)

Paraphilic Disorders

C. Origins
- An assortment of theories have been presented for the origins of paraphilias; however, one has not, as yet, been identified as the true origin. Some suggested origins are:
  - An impulse control disorder, an obsessive-compulsive disorder, or a combination of the two
  - Changes in norepinephrine, serotonin, and dopamine that can change a person's sexual appetite, impulsivity, compulsivity, and antisocial behaviors
  - Excessive testosterone
  - An interruption in the normal courtship phase[5]
  - Distortion of a child's love maps during the vulnerable ages of 5 to 8 years as a result of vandalization[6]
  - Prenatal developmental issues associated with maternal estrogen levels
  - It has been suggested that all humans may have limited paraphilic tendencies (toward continuation of the species) that non-paraphilic people suppress and control (source unknown)

"Paraphilias range from playful and harmless to bizarre and deadly."

— John Money

D. Background
- Treatment for a paraphilia or a paraphilic disorder has improved considerably over the past 20 years; consequently, the prognosis for control and management (but not cure) is positive
- People (usually men) do not seek help for their paraphilic behavior until they have no other choice, e.g., arrested, lost job, relationships
- Prevalence is extremely difficult to determine because these individuals do not trust healthcare professionals with their information; they are especially reluctant to discuss their disorder since many of the activities of paraphilias are illegal as well as socially shunned
- More people with paraphilias live and work within the sex media, pornography, and sex paraphernalia industries than are found within the healthcare environment
- Paraphilias are usually established by age 18, many offenses occur in early adulthood, and few cases over age 50 years are seen (except for pedophilia)[7]
- Male patients with pedophilia, voyeurism, and exhibitionism are seen most frequently in sexual clinics, and men with sexual sadism and sexual masochism are seen least frequently
- It is emphasized by APA[2] that most people with unusual sexual practices do not have a mental disorder, and a

paraphilia itself does not warrant a psychiatric diagnosis
- Paraphilic sexual disorders are not socially acceptable forms of sexual expression, are mostly illegal, and occur most frequently in Caucasian men

E. Therapeutic Interventions
- Perform a Standard Sexual Assessment (Appendix C) and medical assessment, and obtain sexual and medical histories
- The treatment goals for a person with a paraphilia or a paraphilic disorder are to reduce or remove inappropriate sexual arousal behaviors and increase appropriate sexual arousal behaviors, as well as reduce the personal distress associated with the paraphilic disorder. Consequently, many of the same therapeutic interventions are used for different paraphilic disorders, regardless of the offending stimulus for the paraphilia
- Consider the possibility of multiple paraphilias
- Complete the Abel screen for interest in paraphilias and phallometric tumescence testing, or penile strain gauge testing[3]
- Complete all routine preliminary screening of patient's blood—chemistry levels, immune system levels, hormone levels, existence of STIs, HIV, and/or hepatitis
- Determine diagnostic procedures needed, to include electroencephalogram, computerized tomography, and

magnetic resonance imaging evaluations according to physical and history findings[3]
- Determine consultation referrals needed, especially a psychiatrist, psychologist, or a mental health nurse practitioner competent in the management of a person with a paraphilic disorder; a social worker; and a medical physician skilled in the treatment of STDs, HIV, and hepatitis, among others
- Cognitive Behavioral Therapy (CBT), together with Relapse Prevention, has been the mainstay of treatment for paraphilias for many years, and clinical reports support its efficacy. However, some specialists have found that the evidence to support this therapy is weak, and more research is needed[8]
- CBT includes modification of distorted thinking and cognitive restructuring, orgasmic reconditioning, masturbatory satiation, boredom, and extinction; covert sensitization, systematic desensitization, victim empathy, and risk management; relapse and re-relapse prevention; and sex education (Appendix D)
- Pharmacological interventions include SSRIs to increase the serotonin level; medications to reduce emotional conditions, anxiety, depression, obsessive-compulsive disorder symptoms; and anti-androgens to reduce testosterone.
- Stress management techniques, assertiveness skills training,

and social skills rehabilitation
- A number of combination treatment therapies are used; one approach suggested by McDonald[9] and Bradford includes a tiered or levels program:
  - **Level/all levels** - Cognitive Behavioral Therapy and relapse prevention
  - **Level 2** - SSRIs to increase the serotonin level and control depression
  - **Level 3** - Medroxyprogesterone (MPA) to increase elimination of testosterone luteinizing releasing hormone (LRH)
  - **Level 4** - Cyproterone (CPA) an oral antiandrogen and antigonadotropic, or MPA orally daily
  - **Level 5** - MPA intramuscularly (IM) weekly or CPA IM every two weeks
  - **Level 6** - Complete androgen suppression and sex drive suppression (person will be asexual) through use of CPA or LRH IM weekly
- Surgical interventions such as bilateral orchidectomy (surgical castration) or chemical castration for sexual conditions are rarely performed today

F. Supportive Interventions
- Review the Supportive Interventions Guide for Adults (Appendix H)

- Obtain modified sexual and medical history
- Discuss the patient's paraphilic sexual behaviors; his feelings, fears, and concerns
- Monitor for potential substance abuse, mood disorders, and STIs
- Monitor medications for compliance and positive and/or negative effects
- Provide sex education
- Reinforce relapse prevention methods and monitor for re-relapse potential
- Determine which medical interventions have been prescribed, and monitor and assist accordingly. Especially determine any adverse effects of SSRIs as they tend to inhibit orgasm
- Never condone any illegal sexual activity, and do not permit patient to use his distress as an excuse for his behavior

G. Potential Outcomes
- There is no known cure for a paraphilia or a paraphilic disorder; however, motivated patients may see increased calm with a reduction in urges and distress with current interventions; prognosis is better than 20 years ago
- Recent treatments protocols have seen improvement in outcomes, and control of a paraphilia is not unreachable
- Positive outcomes may occur when the patient complies with therapy, has other sexual outlets, has just one paraphilia, and had a later age of onset

- Negative outcomes may occur when the patient is uncooperative with therapy; secretive, and untruthful, has other paraphilias, has no regard for his victims or his family, and had an early age of onset

"The term paraphilia is derived from two Greek words 'para' and 'philia;' 'para' means outside of, and 'philia' means friendship or love. Also referred to as 'beyond normal'."

— John Money

2. Eight Paraphilias and Paraphilic Disorders Identified and Described by APA's DSM-5

Eight paraphilias[2] (exhibitionistic disorder, fetishistic disorder, frotteuristic disorder, pedophilic disorder, sexual masochistic disorder, sexual sadistic disorder, transvestic disorder, and voyeuristic disorder) were selected by DSM-5 for descriptions of symptoms and management for two main reasons. First, "they are relatively common in relationship to other paraphilic disorders," and second, "some of them entail actions for their satisfaction that, because of their noxiousness or potential harm to others, are classed as criminal offenses."[10 (p1)]

DSM-5 also identifies other categories that do not fulfill the two criteria noted above.

i) Exhibitionistic Paraphilia and Disorder

A. Definitions

- **A₁. Exhibitionism Paraphilia Definition**: Over a period of at least six months, recurrent and intense sexual fantasies, sexual urges, or sexual behavior involving the exposure of one's genitals to an unsuspecting stranger[1]

- **A₂. Exhibitionistic Disorder Definition.** In addition to the exhibitionism paraphilia defined above, the person is distressed or impaired by these attractions, or has sought sexual stimulation from exposing the genitals to three or more unsuspecting strangers on separate occasions.[1]

B. Signs and Symptoms
- Recurrent, impulsive showing of one's genitals to an unsuspecting, usually unwilling person or unwilling audience; the victim's shock or surprise adds to the pleasure
- The shame, guilt, and self-reprisal for the man come after masturbation and orgasm, and lasts until the urges return

- May or may not have associated distress
- Four levels of symptoms for exhibitionism were suggested by DSM-3-R (1987) in Frey[7]
    1. "Mild. The person has recurrent fantasies of exposing himself, but has rarely or never, acted upon them.
    2. Moderate. The person has occasionally exposed himself (three targets or fewer) and has difficulty controlling urges to do so.
    3. Severe. The person exposed himself to more than three people and has serious problems with control.
    4. Catastrophic. This level would not be found in exhibitionists without other paraphilias. This level denotes the presence of sadistic features which, if acted upon, would result in serious injury or death to the victim." [7]
    (Blog,para6)

C. Origins
- May be a disorder of impulse control, an obsessive-compulsive disorder, or a chemical imbalance
- A dysfunctional family environment during childhood or childhood trauma such as abuse
- Origin suggestions also include 1) biological

as testosterone increases the susceptibility of males to develop deviant sexual behaviors; 2) learned behaviors from emotional abuse and family dysfunction in childhood; and 3) psychological, based on the assumption that male gender identity requires a male child's separation from his mother so that he does not identify with her as a member of the same sex[7]
- A connection to ADHD has been noted; the actual connection is unknown, but it is seen in men with multiple paraphilias

D. Background
- Exhibitionism, also referred to as *flashing*, is most often performed by Caucasian men
- Exhibitionism is one of the three most common sexual offenses in police records, together with voyeurism and pedophilia; few exhibitionists are females[7]
- Exhibitionists have the highest recidivism rate of all the paraphilias; 20-50% are re-arrested within 2 years[7]
- Most professionals believe the frequency of exhibitionism is underreported and underdiagnosed
- Exhibitionists usually want no actual physical

Paraphilic Disorders

interaction with the victim, and they always make sure they have a rapid exit route planned
- Chronic unemployment, financial difficulties, and marital and family discord if disorder known by others
- Depression, shame, anger, and despair may be experienced by the man; it is dependent upon his arrest record, loss of control, urges, and frequency of exhibitionism
- The individual may or may not have associated distress
- If caught during exposure, the offender is subject to legal prosecution
- Few women are exhibitionists in the ways described above; instead, they undress in front of windows (especially with the curtains open and a light shining behind), or wear low-cut tops and high-cut skirts, which pass as socially accepted behaviors and thereby satiate their inner urges legitimately

E. Therapeutic Interventions
- Perform a Standard Sexual Assessment (Appendix C) and medical assessment, and obtain a sexual and medical history

- Determine the diagnostic tests according to his physical and expressed findings
- Complete the Abel screen for interest in paraphilias and phallometric tumescence testing, or penile strain gauge testing[3]
- Determine medications to be used and implement as soon as possible as further episodes of exhibitionism are likely
- Growth hormones (GnRH analogues) have become the first approach to reduce sexual interest in specific paraphilic activities
- Treatment time has lessened as psychotherapy is not usually involved
- Evaluate patient for substance and alcohol abuse

F. Supportive Interventions
- Review the Supportive Interventions Guide for Adults (Appendix H)
- Obtain modified sexual and medical history, and discuss the patient's paraphilic sexual behaviors; his feelings, fears, and concerns
- Discuss his physical and emotional responses to his mode of therapy, and monitor test results
- Monitor for potential substance abuse, mood disorders, and STIs

- Monitor medications for compliance and positive and/or negative effects
- Provide sex education
- Reinforce relapse prevention methods and monitor for re-relapse potential
- Determine which medical interventions have been prescribed, and monitor and assist accordingly

G. Potential Outcomes
- Some response occurs to medications and CBT (especially covert sensitization), but only if treatments are consistent and maintained
- Some recidivism can be reduced but remains high for many exhibitionists
- The *catastrophic* level indicates the potential for sadistic fantasies, which, without treatment, may result in serious injuries or even death to the victim/stranger

ii) Fetishistic Disorder

A. Definitions.

A_1 Fetishism Paraphilia Definition. The patient

experiences recurrent and intense sexual arousal (manifested by fantasies, urges, or behaviors) either from the use of nonliving objects or from a highly specific focus on non-genital body parts; symptoms must be present for at least six months.[1]

A₂. Fetishistic Paraphilic Disorder Definition. In addition to the fetishistic paraphilia defined above, the patient experiences significant distress or impairment in social, occupational, or other important areas of functioning because of the fantasies, urges, or behaviors. The fetishes are not limited to articles of female clothing used in cross-dressing (as in transvestic disorder) or devices[1]

B. Signs and Symptoms
- May have a body part fetish, most frequently of the feet, hands, and hair (partialism, specifically a non-sexual part[13]) or an object fetish; most frequently of shoes, gloves, and underwear (preferably soiled panties). The man smells, holds/touches, or rubs the object against his genitals
- Masturbation may take place if partner is present or not; however, the object must be present for excitement and arousal to take place. Erectile

Paraphilic Disorders

  dysfunction may occur if the object is not available
- Significant interpersonal difficulties, especially marital, may be present
- The shame, guilt, and self-reprisal for the man come after masturbation and orgasm, and last until the urges return
- Many may not have any distress associated with the fetishism and believe they are not harming selves or others; consequently, they do not believe their fetishistic behavior warrants being called a paraphilia, nor that they have a mental condition
- Condition has been seen in boys as young as four years of age

C. Origins
- Fetishes can be a non-clinical manifestation of a normal spectrum of eroticism causing significant interpersonal difficulties, or may be relaxing rather than arousing[13]
- Early imprinting and conditioning, where excitement and orgasm were associated with a non-sexual object, have also been suggested as origins for fetishes
- Fetishism, transvestism, homosexuality, attention-deficit/hyperactivity disorder, obsessive-

compulsive disorder, and kleptomania may all be linked[13]

D. Background
- Attraction to the feet of women by men is suggested to be more prevalent than their attraction to female breasts
- Frequency rates for fetishism vary. Abel[14] found that 3.4% of his study of 361 men with a paraphilia had fetishism, while in his study of 859 male persons with a paraphilia, just 12 were diagnosed with fetishism. Darcangelo[15] found in her study of approximately 5,000 men that 33% had a foot fetish, and 30% had a fetish for foot-related objects; the remainder were for observation of sexual behaviors of self and others
- The fetish objects used by homosexual men are usually masculine
- Men rarely seek medical treatment; either embarrassment or shame preclude sharing; they do not feel their fetishism is an issue for them or do not want to change
- Fetishism is rarely dangerous to the person or others; consequently, fetishists resent their sexual interest being classified as a paraphilia
- Considered to be a variation of normal sexual

behavior and is tolerated by society, although not usually by a man's female sex partner
- A heterosexual and homosexual activity

E. Therapeutic Interventions
- People rarely seek a physician's help as they do not consider their fetishistic behavior to be abnormal; usually do not want to relinquish fetishistic activities
- Perform a Standard Sexual Assessment (Appendix C) and medical assessment, and obtain sexual and medical histories
- If treatment sought, it includes CBT (especially orgasmic reconditioning, covert sensitization), and occasionally hypnosis
- Prescribe SSRIs, GnRh, antiandrogens according to need
- Complete the Abel screen for interest in paraphilias, and phallometric tumescence testing, or penile strain gauge testing[3]
- Determine level of sexual knowledge and teach to areas of need

F. Supportive Interventions
- Review the Supportive Interventions Guide for Adults (Appendix H)

- People rarely seek supportive assistance from HCPs
- Monitor for adverse effects of medications if prescribed
- Monitor any treatment for positive and negative impact
- Provide sex education
- Provide support and counseling to female partner of heterosexual man

G. Potential Outcomes
- Most enjoy their fetishistic behavior, whether alone or accompanied; however, it is not an activity that they verbally share with many others
- Rarely is a person with fetishistic behavior accused of this as an illegal activity

iii) Frotteuristic Disorder

A. Definitions.

A_1 **Definition of Frotteurism Paraphilia:** The patient experiences recurrent and intense sexual arousal (manifested by fantasies, urges, or behaviors) that involves touching and rubbing against a non-consenting person;

symptoms must be present for at least six months.[1]

A₂. Definition of Frotteuristic Disorder: In addition to the defined frotteurism ("frotteur" is French for *one who rub*s) paraphilia above: The patient experiences significant distress or impairment in social, occupational, or other important areas of functioning because of the fantasies, urges, or behaviors, or the patient has acted on the sexual urges.[1]

B. Signs and Symptoms
- Individual chooses a crowded place (with an exit strategy), and rubs up against or touches the non-consenting, unsuspecting woman who is usually not sure whether this is actually purposeful rubbing. He usually does not look at the woman in the pretense that he is not rubbing up against her
- The shame, guilt, and self-reprisal for the man come after masturbation and orgasm, and remain until the urges return
- May ejaculate into material wrapped around his penis or directly onto the woman
- May or may not have associated distress
- Women either do not recognize the act for what it is, and usually do not speak out about it

C. Origins
- As with other paraphilias, the cause or origin is unknown
- May have been accidental the first time and that episode resulted in arousal, so pattern is repeated
- May have been sexually assaulted as a child
- May have a lack of impulse control
- May be a case of courtship disorder

D. Background
- Person is a little older, considered to be a loner, shy, and introverted
- Activities begin around age 15-25
- Frotteurist seeks crowded places for his frotteuristic behavior, usually on public transport during the rush hour
- If detected, he usually claims accidental touching
- People may not recognize the frotteurism, or they ignore the frotteuristic activity
- Rarely visits a psychologist or counselor
- Has problems with authorities; questionable if as a result of frotteurism or occurred before
- His behavior causes alarm in his victim, but does not cause physical harm

Paraphilic Disorders

E. Therapeutic Interventions
- Perform a Standard Sexual Assessment (Appendix C) and medical assessment, and obtain a sexual and medical history
- Complete the Abel screen for interest in paraphilias and phallometric tumescence testing, or penile strain gauge testing[3]
- As with other paraphilias, certain aspects of CBT are used, especially orgasmic reconditioning
- Advise to implement distractive techniques such as music, reading, sports, etc. when urges arise
- Twelve-step programs relating to, or characteristic of a program that is designed to help an individual overcome an addiction, compulsion, serious sexual shortcoming, or traumatic experience by adherence to 12 tenets emphasizing personal growth and dependence on a higher spiritual being (Appendix D)
- Prescribe GnRH analogues or Medroxyprogesterone to reduce sexual desire and arousal, SSRIs if depressed
- Determine presence of poor social skills and implement interventions such as assertiveness skills training, conversation skills, intimacy skills, social skills

F. Supportive Interventions
- Review the Supportive Interventions Guide for Adults (Appendix H)
- Reinforce CBT
- Reinforce acquisition and practice of new social skills
- Support activities of distraction to abort his urges
- Monitor for signs of relapse
- Monitor the effects of Medroxyprogesterone, SSRIs, GnRH analogues

G. Potential Outcomes
- Treatment may change the person's frotteuristic behaviors to more socially acceptable ones, if the man continues therapy and if he adheres to the treatment program
- Usually remains a chronic condition; may be arrested if detected
- Success determined by man's desire to change
- If court-ordered treatment, the prognosis is usually not positive

iv) Pedophilic Disorder

A. Definitions

A₁. Definition of Pedophilic Paraphilia: The man reports recurrent and intense sexually arousing fantasies, sexual urges, or behaviors involving sexual activity with a prepubescent child or children (generally less than or equal to 13 years); symptoms must be present for at least six months[1]

A₂. Definition of Pedophilic Disorder: In addition to the defined pedophilic paraphilia above, the disorder causes great distress or interpersonal difficulty within the offender, or the individual has acted on his sexual urges. The individual is age at least 16 years and at least five years older than the victim; individuals in late adolescence involved in an ongoing sexual relationship with a 12 or 13 year old are excluded[1]

B. Signs and Symptoms
- Pedophiles are defined by their desires, rather than their behavior, and not all pedophiles act upon their desires. Some pedophiles never have any sexual activity with a child, but it is difficult to determine in

what numbers this occurs; however, they spend their lives experiencing extreme anxiety about the sexual urges they have toward children and fear what they might be tempted to do to a child

- Pedophiles have abnormal and unnatural sexual and physical attractions toward children (usually prepubescent and under age 13) that result in anxiety, guilt, and difficulties in pursuing and achieving their life goals; their urges cause them to approach children for actual sexual gratification

- Pedophiles have various levels of sexual activities with their young victims, and they usually increase the level of child sexual intrusion slowly and carefully. They may begin by looking at pictures of a naked child, then actually looking at the naked child, then masturbating in front of the child, then touching a child non-sexually, and then touching sexually, rubbing genitals against the child, then asking the child to touch his genitals, performing oral sex, then penetrative sex (mostly when children are older)

- The pedophile may have marked distress associated with his pedophilic behavior; however, this distress is often accompanied by unbelievable, lengthy, and convoluted justifications for that same behavior. A U.S. Justice Manual for law officers identifies five common defense patterns in pedophiles:

(1) Denial ("Is it wrong to give a child a hug?")

(2) Minimization ("It only happened once")

(3) Justification ("I am a boy lover, not a child molester")

(4) Fabrication (activities were for research for a scholarly project)

(5) Attack (character attacks on the child, prosecutors, or police, as well as potential for physical violence)[16]

- The majority of pedophiles have at least one other paraphilia such as frotteurism, voyeurism, exhibitionism, or sadism
- As the pedophile's stress level increases, so does his frequency of offenses
- Often associated with other psychological issues

C. Origins
- As with other paraphilias, the exact cause is unknown
- Some theories proposed for origin include:
  - Environmental or psychosocial factors such as sexual or physical abuse and neglect as a child
  - Inability to develop close relationships with adults, and failure to reach adult maturity
  - The man's interaction with his parents when he was a young child, perhaps with a religious, patriarchal upbringing

- The need for the man to have a non-dominating sexual partner, one whom the pedophile can dominate
- Left home at an early age due to poverty, alcoholism, lack of warmth in the family
- Hormonal influences from maternal stress while offender is in-utero, with an increase in maternal steroids, and an excess of testosterone

D. Background
- Approximately 1% of all men 17-80 years of age are considered to be pedophiles, and they mostly offend in their later years, ages 40-70.[17] Pedophilic disorder is far more common among men than women
- Coercion or force is rarely needed to get the child to comply with the pedophile; the pedophile has gained the child's trust through seduction, manipulation, and convincing lies. This trust relationship is achieved through what is known as the *grooming* of the child phase
- The pedophile may also be very personable and likeable to the child; he may be a friendly volunteer, someone who spends time with the child, a professional helper, a relative, someone who is patient and very good with children

Paraphilic Disorders

- Pedophiles may have an attraction to boys and girls, or have an attraction toward boys or girls only, or they are attracted both to adults and children
- Pedophilia is one of the most common paraphilias, together with voyeurism and exhibitionism

E. Therapeutic Interventions
- Perform a Standard Sexual Assessment (Appendix C) and medical assessment, and obtain sexual and medical histories
- Complete the Abel screen for interest in paraphilias and phallometric tumescence testing, or penile strain gauge testing[3]
- Obtain specialty consultations (as needed) such as marriage and family therapist, pediatric nurse practitioner or pediatric psychologist (for the abused child), social worker, psychologist or psychiatrist, drug dependency therapist, pharmacologist, group therapy leader
- Cognitive-behavioral and relapse prevention programs in North America have been the predominant theories guiding treatment in North America. Components of CBT[8 (p292-3)] include:
    - "Cognitive re-structuring to manage cognitive distortions

- Orgasmic re-conditioning
- Covert sensitization and aversive conditioning
- Masturbatory satiation to make deviant behavior boring
- Systematic de-sensitization to decrease maladaptive anxiety
- Assertiveness skills training to increase ability to express feelings and reduce passive-aggressive approach
- Social skills training
- Sexual education
- Sexual dysfunction treatment
- Empathy therapy toward his victims and apologies to victims (may reduce personal guilt; however, cannot undo the damage done to the victims)
- Personal victimization therapy for the offender
- Therapeutic confrontation therapy and group therapy
- Bibliotherapy, talk therapy, and role-playing
- Eliminate ingestion of drugs, alcohol, high emotions, anger, and marital discord because these contribute to relapse and re-relapse
- Prescribe SSRIs such as sertraline, fluoxetine, fluvoxamine, and paroxetine to inhibit serotonin reuptake; tricyclic antidepressants such as imipramine and desipramine to inhibit serotonin reuptake; lithium to

enhance serotonin function; and medroxytestosterone to inhibit "testosterone"[16(p2)]
- Advise to avoid any interactions alone with children; do not get a job where contact with children is possible

F. Supportive Interventions
- Review the Supportive Interventions Guide for Adults (Appendix H)
- Advise offender regarding his mental health, job, income, and financial security loss; isolation and withdrawal from partner, children, family, and friends
- Administer and monitor medications
- Monitor for illegal drug and alcohol use
- Implement supporting aspects associated with CBT, to include:
  - Support during identification of his cognitive distortions, and re-enforce, firmly, non-use of excuses that support his distortions
  - Discussion of the impact on him if has been sexually abused as a child, but do not support its potential adverse impact as an excuse
  - Continuation of masturbatory satiation techniques when man demonstrates resistance or disinterest until reaches desired level of boredom
  - Provision of social skills examples, especially those

identified by the man as a need
- Provision of sexual education to correct inaccurate information
- Provision of sexual education if sexual dysfunction present

G. Potential Outcomes
- Can never be cured, but can have urges and associated distress reduced with treatment
- Pedophiles rarely seek professional help voluntarily; professional help is usually mandated by the legal system when the pedophile has been caught and charged. If court mandate is the case, popular treatment is CBT, often with a relatively high failure and recidivism rate
- If the pedophile voluntarily seeks treatment for his urges, then there is a slight improvement in the outcomes, but residual effects of the pedophilic behaviors remain
- Most people who have been victimized by a pedophile do not become pedophiles themselves
- Boys and youth who are pedophiles and receive therapy have more positive outcomes from treatment than adult pedophiles. However, if untreated, the incidents escalate, urges do not stop, and the pedophilic activities become chronic

Points for Discussion:

Is the sexual misconduct of a sexual offender a psychological disorder that requires treatment or an antisocial behavior that requires punishment?

v) **Sexual Masochism Disorder and Sexual Sadism Disorders**

DSM-5 (the publication used by mental health professionals as a guide to diagnose and treat mental disorders of patients) was updated in May, 2013, and contained some wording changes in the definitions and criteria of some paraphilic disorders. However, these changes did not alleviate the concerns of most members of the bondage, discipline, sadism, masochism (BDSM) community who feel their unusual sexual activities do not warrant being included in DSM-5[1] as they consider their sexual activities to be consensual and safe. They also resent non-criminal, consensual unusual sex practices (sexual masochism, sexual sadism, transvestism, fetishism) being classified alongside criminal unusual sex practice.

A. **Definitions**

A_1. **Definition of Sexual Masochism Paraphilia:** The patient experiences recurrent and intense sexual arousal (manifested by fantasies, urges, and sexual behaviors) involving the act (real, not simulated) of being humiliated, beaten, bound, or otherwise made to suffer; symptoms must be present for at least six months[1]

A_2. **Definition of a Sexual Masochism Disorder:** In addition to the paraphilia defined above, the fantasies, urges, or behaviors cause significant distress or impairment in social, occupational, or other important areas of functioning[1]

B. **Signs and Symptoms**
- The individual, usually a man, experiences sexual arousal and pleasure from being placed in a position of humiliation (usually by a woman), dressed in clothes appropriate to their desired roles, with sexual paraphernalia necessary to inflict pain and fulfill the man's desired and requested humiliation
- This humiliation-gratifying behavior comes in many diverse forms, either self-inflicted (self-flagellation, cutting, cigarette burning), or inflicted by another, with both engaged in role-playing (slave/master/dominatrix, schoolboy/teacher). May involve being spanked, whipped, handcuffed, tied, chained,

electric shocks, etc.
- An individual may self-flagellate for other reasons than masochism; as a penance for sins, or to demonstrate loyalty
- Shame, guilt, or self-reprisal may or may not occur, but if they do, they come after masturbation and orgasm, and last until the urges return
- May have significant distress or none at all
- Wants to escape from his current world to one that is entirely different
- Hypoxyphilia is an extremely rare and dangerous form of masochism during which a man ties a noose or a tie around his neck, or places a bag over his head to reduce oxygen in an attempt to induce a greater orgasm

C. Origins
- No universally accepted origin has been identified
- Inappropriate sexual fantasies are suppressed, which increases sexual urges, and the masochistic behavior then becomes linked to sexual behavior[19]
- May want to be in the dominating role; becomes confused and anxious and takes subservient role
- Sexual fantasies of a person may have been suppressed by the rigidity of the family or the

community, so the person seeks fulfillment of his fantasies beyond this confinement, which leads to confusion and distress, and to a positive association between pain and sex

D. Background
- Actual prevalence is difficult to estimate as mostly private activity. Some say occurs 20 times more prevalently with men than women, while others say just slightly more prevalent
- As grow older, participation diminishes; very few after age 50
- First noticed in childhood, but begins in early adulthood; not a rare occurrence, with masochism occurring more frequently than sadism
- Participating individuals are expected to have a safety plan in place to reduce harm potential
- Need for psychological humiliation and degradation usually involved

E. Therapeutic Interventions
- Perform a Standard Sexual Assessment (Appendix C) and medical assessment, and obtain sexual and medical histories
- Complete the Abel screen for interest in paraphilias

Paraphilic Disorders

and phallometric tumescence testing, or penile strain gauge testing[3]
- CBT is the treatment of choice, to include cognitive restructuring, reduction of violent behaviors, and promotion of healthy behaviors
- Social skills training
- Determine whether distress is present. If so, prescribe one or more pharmacological interventions according to need. These include SSRIs to increase the serotonin level, phenothiazines to control mental and emotional disorders, and mood stabilizers to prevent intense mood shifts from depression to a manic stage in bipolar disorder; chlomipramine to reduce obsessive-compulsive disorder symptoms; and anti-androgens to reduce testosterone
- Prescribe family or couple therapy if indicated
- Monitor for STIs and treat if present
- If absolutely essential as a sexual stimulus, refer for sex therapy and/or psychiatric therapy
- Monitor for medical conditions that could be a result of the masochism; examples are bone fractures, soft tissue injuries, organ injury, skin breakdown, and infection

F. Supportive Interventions
- Review the Supportive Interventions Guide for Adults (Appendix H)
- Monitor the medical conditions that could be a result of masochism; examples are bone fractures, soft tissue injuries, organ injury, skin breakdown, and infection, among others
- Observe for the potential for blood exchange, and STIs
- Determine whether distress is present and refer to a psychiatric expert if needed
- Support family therapy/partner therapy
- Administer and monitor effects of medications

G. Potential Outcomes
- May become fixated with fantasies of sexual masochism to the point that all family, work, social, and friend relationships are ignored, or the person may reach an acceptable level of excitement that causes him no problems at all and satiates his sexual need
- Significant distress impacts all aspects of man's life
- Interpersonal issues with partner if he or she does not agree with, support, or condone masochistic behavior

- The individual may move into the sexual masochism community life where he may or may not adopt the life
- Older than about age 50 tends to stop masochistic activities

vi) Sexual Sadism Paraphilia and Sexual Sadism Disorder

  A. Definitions

  A_1 **Definition of Sexual Sadism Paraphilia:** The patient experiences recurrent and intense fantasies, urges, or behaviors) from the psychological or physical suffering inflicted on another person; symptoms must be present for at least six months.[1]

  A_2 **Definition of Sexual Sadism Disorder:**
In addition to the sexual sadism paraphilia above, the fantasies, urges, or behaviors cause significant distress or impairment in social, occupational, or other important areas of functioning, or the patient has acted on these sexual urges with a non-consenting person.[1]

  B. Signs and Symptoms
- Sexual excitement obtained from administering pain, humiliation, and embarrassment to another

person, who is most often known to the sadist, but may be unknown
- Sadism with a misjudged sadistic act leading to extreme violence or death of a victim
- Some participants feel there is nothing to be shamed or distressed about as the sexual activities that take place between two adults in their own home are private and consensual
- However, acts may be carried out with non-consenting and unsuspecting individuals; acts that may include quite violent behaviors for which the intended victim may be ill-prepared
- May or not have associated distress because of the sexual sadism
- Shame, guilt, and self-reprisal for the man come after masturbation and orgasm and last until the urges return
- The behaviors begin innocently enough, but advance into more complicated, bizarre sadistic activities

C. Origins
- Brain injuries or mental illnesses such as schizophrenia, antisocial personality
- An individual's need to escape from a life that does not excite

- Sexual fantasies of a person may have been suppressed by the rigidity of the family or the community, so the person seeks fulfillment of his fantasies beyond this confinement, which leads to confusion and distress, and to a positive association between pain and sex

D. Background
- The feelings of power obtained from sexual sadism are claimed to be invigorating and releasing, and individuals who experience a boring life may derive pleasure through a different partner with masochistic needs
- Participating individuals are expected to have a safety plan in place to reduce harm potential
- Probably begins in adolescence
- Participants do not see sadism as a mental nor criminal disorder, and feel it is a behavior between two consenting adults
- The acts are real, not simulated

E. Therapeutic Interventions
- Perform a Standard Sexual Assessment (Appendix C) and medical assessment, and obtain sexual and medical histories

- Complete the Abel screen for interest in paraphilias and phallometric tumescence testing, or penile strain gauge testing[3]
- CBT is the treatment of choice, together with cognitive restructuring, to reduce violent behaviors and promote healthy behaviors
- Determine whether other psychiatric conditions present. If so, prescribe one or more pharmacological interventions according to diagnosis.
- Monitor for STIs and treat if present

F. Supportive Interventions
- Review the Supportive Interventions Guide for Adults (Appendix H)
- Observe for signs of excessive skin breaks and infection
- Observe for the potential for blood exchange, and STIs
- Determine whether distress is present and defer to a psychiatric expert
- If masochism is essential as a sexual stimulus, support sex therapy and/or psychiatric therapy
- Support family therapy/partner therapy
- Administer and monitor effects of medications

G. Potential Outcomes
- The individual may move into the sexual sadism community life where he may or may not adopt the life of a person within the masochism community
- May become fixated with fantasies of sexual sadism to the point that all family, work, social, and friend relationships are ignored, or the person may reach an acceptable level of excitement that causes him no problems at all and satiates his sexual need
- Significant distress impacts all aspects of man's life
- Interpersonal issues with partner when she does not agree with/support/condone his need for his sadistic behavior.
- Older than about age 50, the man tends to stop his activities

vii) Transvestic Fetishism Paraphilia and Disorder

A. Definitions

A₁. Definition of Transvestic Fetishism Paraphilia: The patient experiences recurrent and intense sexual arousal manifested by fantasies, urges, or behaviors from cross-dressing; symptoms must be present for at least six months.[1]

A₁. **Definition of a Transvestic Fetishism Disorder:** In addition to the above, the fantasies, urges, or behaviors cause significant distress or impairment in social, occupational, or other important areas of functioning.[1]

B. **Signs and Symptoms**
- Individual is aroused by the feel of fabrics, materials, or garments (transvestic fetishism), and seeks stimulation from them on an intermittent basis rather than all the time
- May be aroused by thoughts or images of self as female (autogynephilia)
- The individual, most often a heterosexual or bisexual male, may experience shame, guilt, and self-reprisal after masturbation and orgasm, that lasts until the urges return
- May or may not have associated distress, and may or may not have gender identity issues
- Interpersonal issues where the partner does not support the cross-dressing nor the transvestic activities for her partner's sexual arousal

C. **Origins**
- No known identified cause
- Perhaps childhood trauma such as child sex abuse

- Neurological/chemical imbalance
- Dressed in girl's clothes by older females when a child
- Excessive maternal estrogen level while boy in utero

D. Background
- The activity of cross-dressing, previously thought to be preferred only by heterosexual and bisexual males, now includes lesbian women and gay males
- Transvestism is not an illegal act, and it is not considered to be a mental disorder by many
- Fetishism involves inanimate objects, whereas transvestic fetishism involves sexual arousal of one person by another person wearing the clothing of the opposite sex (usually a female), to include bras, underpants, stocking, shoes, and boots. The man loves the touch, feel, and smell of the object, using as many of his senses as possible
- Many men who are transvestites are heterosexual, in a long-time heterosexual relationship, and may or may not masturbate while wearing the other person's clothes; if they wear clothes for sexual arousal and ejaculation, it is considered to be a paraphilia
- Interest in these items of clothing usually begins

around puberty in boys, as do other paraphilias
- Some women are supportive of partner's activities, others are not; they reject the need for the activities for their partner's sexual arousal
- Considered pathological if sexual arousal not obtained without transvestic behaviors, or causes significant distress for the man

E. **Therapeutic Interventions**
- Perform a Standard Sexual Assessment (Appendix C) and medical assessment, and obtain sexual and medical histories
- Complete diagnostic procedures and questionnaires according to existence of other paraphilia or medical condition potential
- Complete the Abel screen for interest in paraphilias and phallometric tumescence testing, or penile strain gauge testing[3]
- Many transvestite individuals do not want to stop their transvestic behaviors; however, his partner may be the reason medical help is sought; consequently, the man is often an unwilling and uncooperative patient
- Refer to partner and family counseling expert for partner/marital/family therapy

- Refer to psychiatrist or mental health nurse practitioner for CBT with orgasmic restructuring
- Evaluate for medication need to support therapy

F. Supportive Interventions
- Review the Supportive Interventions Guide for Adults (Appendix H)
- Determine whether distress is present and confer with psychiatrist or mental health nurse practitioner
- When transvestic behaviors are essential for sexual stimulus and arousal, discuss sex therapy and/or psychiatric therapy interventions, and monitor progress
- Administer and monitor medications

G. Potential Outcomes
- The prognosis is moderate for cessation of transvestic activities if that is what he needs; however, some men do not want to stop as it is not an issue for them (and often brings them great pleasure), so treatment fails
- Relationships may either adapt to the transvestic activities and both partners are content, or the relationship continues acrimoniously, grudgingly, or the relationship ends

viii) Voyeuristic Disorders

A. Definitions

A₁. Definition of Voyeurism Paraphilia: "The patient experiences recurrent and intense sexual arousal (expressed through fantasies, urges or behaviors) involving the act of observing an unsuspecting person who is naked, in the process of disrobing, or engaging in sexual activity; symptoms must be present for at least 6 months"[1]

A₂. Definition of a Voyeuristic Paraphilic Disorder: In addition to the voyeurism paraphilia above, the fantasies, urges, or behaviors cause significant distress or impairment in social, occupational, or other important areas of functioning, or the patient has acted on these urges with a non-consenting person[1]

B. Signs and Symptoms
- Usually hidden from sight, the man watches strangers engaged in sexual activities (a *Peeping Tom*), or a person undressing with the hope that the voyeur can surprise or startle the victim, or a person in the nude
- He may use binoculars, cameras, video cameras to assist visibility
- He may also fantasize that he is sexually arousing the victim while becoming aroused himself

- The shame, guilt, depression, and self-reprisal for the man come after masturbation and orgasm, and remain until the urges return
- May or may not have associated distress and depression
- Employment issues, financial issues, interpersonal and intrapersonal issues prevail, especially with his partner
- Does not seek physical contact with his victim(s)

C. Origins
- No known cause or origin
- May be associated with conditioning or imprinting from childhood
- One suggestion is that a child or young man inadvertently witnesses the genitals of a person, or a nude person, or people making love when he is young, and he interprets his feelings to be sexual. He repeatedly fantasizes until the voyeurism becomes a requirement for his sexual arousal

D. Background
- Condition usually presents itself before age 15[20]
- Individual rarely seeks medical help voluntarily, usually occurs with a court order as voyeurism is a criminal act

E. Therapeutic Interventions
- Perform a Standard Sexual Assessment (Appendix C) and medical assessment, and obtain sexual and medical histories
- Treatment is usually mandated by the court, so the man is an unwilling participant in any interventions
- Complete the Abel screen for interest in paraphilias and phallometric tumescence testing, or penile strain gauge testing[3]
- Refer to a psychiatrist, sexologist, or mental health nurse practitioner for CBT to perhaps change voyeuristic behaviors to behaviors that are more healthy and socially acceptable
- No specific medications can cure voyeurism, but may modify behavior
- Prescribe medications such as SSRIs to increase the serotonin level and reduce depression, phenothiazines to control serious mental and emotional disorders, chlomipramine to reduce obsessive-compulsive disorder symptoms, and antiandrogens to reduce testosterone

F. Supportive Interventions
- Review the Supportive Interventions Guide for Adults (Appendix C)

- Determine whether the patient has any depression or distress, and if so, request expert assistance
- Evaluate patient for employment status, financial status, residential status, and the interpersonal issues with important people in his life
- Evaluate if friendless without support

G. Potential Outcomes
- Prognosis is usually not good if voyeurism is the man's only sexual outlet
- Not easy to prosecute as intent is hard to prove
- Embarrassment from being caught in the act might deter
- Voyeurism often persists as a chronic sexual outlet that the man is loath to relinquish, often to the exclusion of all other sexual activities

3. DSM-5 Specified and Unspecified Paraphilic Disorders

Other Specified and Unspecified Paraphilic Disorders identified in DSM-5 are disorders in which symptoms of a paraphilia or paraphilic disorder are present in an individual but they do not meet the two specific DSM-5 criteria as do the eight paraphilic behaviors described earlier. These other paraphilic disorders include:

- **Asphyxophilia** or **Hypoxyphilia** – A potentially

harmful self-inflicted deprivation of oxygen to the brain to enhance sexual arousal and orgasm
- **Coprophilia** – An unnatural arousing interest in feces and their expulsion from the body of self or another
- **Infantilism** - an erotic attraction to infants
- **Klismaphilia** - Sexual gratification obtained by receiving an enema
- **Necrophilia** - Sexual gratification by viewing or having intercourse with a dead body (very rare)
- **Partialism** - Being sexually attracted to a particular part of the body; with "equally or greater erotic attraction than genitals."[15 (p405)]
- **Telephone Scatologia** - Overt or covert repetitive phone calls with non-consenting adults that are sexually obscene
- **Urophilia** - Sexual arousal and orgasm is dependent on urination by one person on another (*golden showers*), or drinking the urine of others, and vice versa
- **Zoophilia** - An erotic fixation on animals that sexually arouses, that may or may not result in intercourse attempts with the animal

4. Other Examples of Paraphilic Disorders

John Money,[6] a prominent psychologist from the 1960s to the

1990s, identified and described over 40 unusual sexual behaviors, some of which are included in DSM-5, others that are not; most are considered to be rare. Some authors claim over 500 paraphilias. As with other paraphilias, some of these unusual sexual behaviors are considered non-harmful, consensual, and non-coercive, while others are not. Some examples include:

- **Acrotomophilia** – A person who becomes sexually aroused and desires a person who has a disability, primarily an amputee
- **Apotemnophilia** – A person who becomes sexually aroused and excited at the thought of self as an amputee
- **Autonepiophilia** – Sexual arousal when treated as and dressed as a baby (in diapers, bottle-fed)
- **Ephebophilia** – Sexual arousal through watching/touching a post-pubescent pre-adult girl or boy
- **Erotophonophilia** – Sexual arousal through the act of killing or the image of killing another person
- **Gerontophilia** – Sexual arousal by a younger person for an elderly man or woman
- **Hibristophilia** – Sexual interest and arousal that occurs in a person (usually a woman) by a person (usually a man) who has committed a robbery, a murder, a rape, or similar act of extreme violence; often incarcerated
- **Kleptophilia** – Sexual arousal by stealing items from another person

- **Mysophilia** – sexual arousal and gratification by touching filthy, sweaty, menses blood-stained or soaked underwear
- **Pictophilia** – Compulsive viewing of sexually graphic pictures that sexually arouse
- **Self-Flagellation** – Self-whipping as a penance or demonstration of loyalty and affiliation
- **Sexuoerotic Age Discrepancy** – A sexual attraction between a very young person and a very old person
- **Somnophilia** – Sexual arousal and urges toward a sleeping, unconscious person
- **Stigmatophilia** – Sexual arousal and pleasure from another person who is marked in some way, i.e., tattoos, scars, body piercings

As can be seen by the descriptions of the paraphilias and paraphilic disorders above, they are not conditions that are easily accepted, managed, or understood. Inexperienced HCPs are encouraged to leave the management of these conditions to those who have the required experience, knowledge, and skills, and are not threatened by the behaviors of the person with a paraphilia. However, some knowledge of these conditions provides inexperienced HCPs a foundation with which they can discuss, assure, and support the person with a paraphilia until which time the HCP, in turn, becomes the expert.

APPENDICES

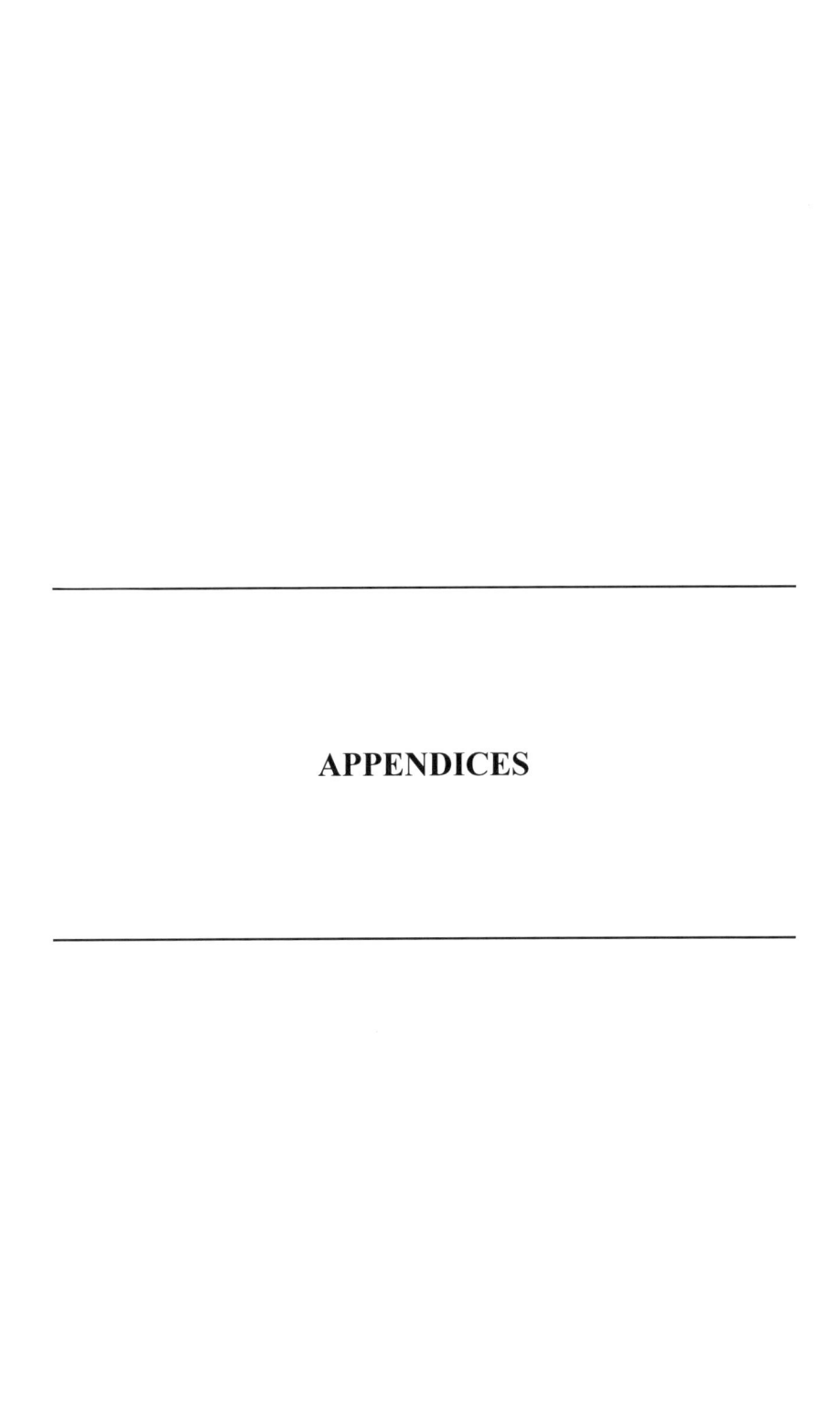

Appendix A
How Comfortable Are You with Your Own Sexuality?
Please Write Down Your First Thoughts
(For Your Eyes Only)

According to Foley, Kope, and Sugrue (2002)[1] when a woman is asked whether she is comfortable with her sexuality, many instinctively answer *yes* until they are asked questions similar to those below...

1. Are you at ease when you undress before your partner?

    Y N N/A

2. Are you at ease when you stand naked in front of a full mirror?

    Y N N/A

3. Are you relaxed during lovemaking?

    Y N N/A

4. Can you find pleasure in tactile sensations without distractions/guilt?   Y N N/A

5. Do you feel completely free to explore your sexuality, try new things?   Y N N/A

6. Do you feel completely free to talk openly with your partner?

    Y N N/A

7. Do you feel confident when educating others about sex?

    Y N N/A

8. Do you have uncertainty about any aspect of your sexuality?

    Y N N/A

9. Are you more conservative sexually than your peers?

    Y N N/A

10. Are you more liberal sexually than your peers?

    Y N N/A

This questionnaire may be responded to by men also.

Appendix B
How Comfortable Are You with Patient Sexuality?
Please Write Down Your First Thoughts

(For Your Eyes Only)

Ask Yourself:

1. Am I comfortable with the sexuality of patients?

    Y N N/A

2. Do I get embarrassed/upset by some patients' sexual behavior?   Y N N/A

3. Do I look a patient directly in the eyes during discussions about sex?   Y N N/A

4. Do I recognize my own limitations during sexual discussions with patients?   Y N N/A

5. Am I able to meet a patient's needs during sexual discussions?

    Y N N/A

6. Do my own views on sexuality impact how I interact with patients?   Y N N/A

7. Do I know when I am out of my depth discussing sexual concerns with patients?   Y N N/A

8. Am I able to answer patients' questions honestly and truthfully?   Y N N/A

9. Am I non-judgmental about a patient's sexual expression?
   Y N N/A

10. Do I act and speak as though I am heterosexist?
    Y N N/A

Appendix C
Standard Sexual Assessment

- Put patient at ease, and inform that a sex history is an important part of a medical history
- Inform that you ask these questions regardless of age, gender, sexual orientation, or marital status, and his/her information is treated with the utmost confidentiality
- Using open-ended yet direct questions, obtain a sexual history, and include the 5 "P"s of sexual health and STDs: Partners, practices, protection from STDs, past history of STDs, and prevention of pregnancy[2]
- Never make assumptions about the patient's sexual orientation, partner status, or sexual activities
- Obtain a past and present sexual history from the individual (involve partner at a later point) to include items such as:
  - sexual experiences during early childhood, puberty, and adulthood
  - childhood home and family environment, and parental attitude toward sexuality
  - current sexual history of personal sexual satisfaction/ dissatisfaction, and discuss specific activities involved, such as fantasy, desire, arousal, erectile function and lubrication, masturbation, preferred sexual outlets, frequency of sexual activities, sexual orientation, sexual dysfunctions (to include current main sexual issue), gender identity dysphoria

- past 12 months number of sex partners and current number, and whether men, women, or both, and time-length of relationship(s)
 - past and present substance abuse history
 - past and present pregnancy and STI risk-reduction methods (monogamy, abstinence, condom use, STI testing, education) and situations when used
 - past and present risky sexual behaviors to include unprotected sex, use of illegal drugs, birth control practices, history of sexual abuse, and illegal sexual activities
- Evaluate accuracy of the individual's sexual knowledge
- Obtain a psychiatric history and examination as some psychiatric issues lead to sexual problems
- Obtain a medical history and perform a medical physical assessment as many medical issues lead to sexual problems
- Administer sexual questionnaires according to specific sexual issue
- Determine which diagnostic tests need to be performed, according to presenting symptoms, and which HCP consultation specialists may need to be involved to manage sexual issues most effectively
- Examples of consultations that may be beneficial include with a cardiologist, endocrinologist, genitourinary surgeon, nurse practitioner, geneticist, physical therapist, psychiatrist, psychologist, sexual transition surgeon, sexologist, sexual therapist, vascular surgeon, and specialist in STIs and HIV

Appendix D
Examples of Therapies and Techniques Applied to Sexual Issues

Cognitive Behavioral Therapy (CBT) has been the mainstay of treatment of sexual issues for many years, as a collection of therapies prescribed for sexual dysfunctions, depression, paraphilias, anorgasmia, orgasm dysfunctions, and anxiety disorders, among others. Rationale for their use is based on the assumption that all behaviors are learned, and focus is on how they can be unlearned rather than the reasons they occur. CBT uses modeling, social skills training, relaxation techniques, problem-solving techniques, and orgasmic reconditioning, among many others.

The therapist and the individual develop a goal-oriented and focused relationship in which they both examine the patient's thoughts and patterns of thought, his feelings in response to those thoughts, and the behaviors that occur as a result. By knowing what precipitates the unwanted behaviors, the goal is to unlearn and modify them, then learn and develop more acceptable behaviors. Can be provided on an individual or group basis dependent upon the sexual condition and the individual's needs.

Coital Positions are of importance in any sexual relationship, and are especially so when one or both partners are incapacitated by illness. Many articles have been written about which position is best to achieve the maximum sexual satisfaction during coitus; however, the primary goal is to achieve sexual satisfaction with the least amount of fatigue, pain, or discomfort; then sexual arousal has a greater opportunity to occur. The main points to remember are to strive for a position in which both partners are fully supported, one that avoids muscle cramping, promotes the best blood flow to the larger muscles, and enhances flexibility. Coital positions and sexual techniques also have to meet with the value systems of both partners.

Couple or Partner Therapy is where two sexual partners meet with an unbiased sexologist, sex therapist, or psychiatrist to discuss the couple's communication issues, interpersonal problems, and sexual concerns, including unhealthy sexual activities, their sexual conflicts, and unwanted sexual triggers. Interventions include negotiation skills, sexual activity assignments, development of mutual respect, active listening, non-interrupting talk, role playing, and behavioral therapy. Partner therapy assists couples in dealing with the multitudes of situations they face on an everyday basis, usually using behavior modification techniques.

Family Therapy is what its name implies. Family members gather in a non-threatening group setting to discuss their conflicts, their inability to address problems, and any unhealthy activities; as well as to recognize and manage their own and relatives' emotions, and practice active listening. An unbiased therapist guides the process.

Group Therapy is where people with similar sexual problems (often those that involve victims) gather in a group setting to discuss their experiences and intervention successes and failures. They take responsibility for their actions and acknowledge the impact on their victims and families; peer support is a cornerstone while an unbiased therapist guides the process.

Interpersonal Psychotherapy does not address the actual issue between two or more people or its cause, but rather focuses on improvement of the interpersonal relationship that exists between an individual and a specific person or persons. It concentrates on issues that are the "genesis of psychiatric distress" for an individual, and is a relatively short time-limited program of approximately 6 to 20 visits,[3] conducted by a psychiatrist or psychologist

Kegel Exercises are conscious, repeated contractions and relaxation of the muscle that comprise part of the pelvic floor, the pubococcygeal muscle. This muscle helps control urinary and defecation activities, and Kegel exercises improve the muscle's tone in preparation for a number of sexual conditions, such as muscle toning to assist before and after childbirth, to reduce premature ejaculation, to increase sexual pleasure, and to tighten prolapse of pelvic floor in women. External devices to aid Kegel exercises do not usually work.

Masturbatory Extinction or Satiation requires that the patient masturbates to orgasm, and then continues to masturbate for

431

one hour after he has reached orgasm. Since there is no orgasm/ejaculation, there is no reward; the goal is masturbatory boredom, and the reduction of interest in masturbation and/or the person's usual fantasies.

Orgasmic Re-Conditioning requires that the patient thinks of his fantasy, describes the fantasy out loud while masturbating, and masturbates to orgasm. Later does the same, but as orgasms, looks at picture of an appropriate partner, either male or female. Repeats this process until only reaches orgasm with an appropriate partner.

Pharmacologic Therapy includes the use of medications to treat conditions such as depression, anxiety, lack of lubrication, arousal and desire issues, erectile dysfunction, orgasm issues, reduced testosterone and estrogen, among others. Often different medications are used to treat the same dysfunction, and HCPs prescribe medications according to their personal experience of each medication's success, knowledge of its use, its efficiency and efficacy, what they were taught in training, and the literature and research study reports.

Relapse Prevention Techniques require a patient to learn how to identify red flags or warnings about the return of unwanted behaviors and to identify and correct those unwanted behaviors. He learns how to ask for help and actually to ask; to give self some other rewards instead of the undesirable reward; to avoid risky situations, places, and behaviors, and to know the positive and negative consequences of any actions taken. Note: a relapse involves just one episode of unwanted behavior, whereas a re-relapse involves repeated unwanted behaviors over a period of time.

Sensate Focus is a process that directs a couple's activities away from sexual performance and coitus toward an increased awareness of the pleasurable feelings associated with their own body and senses. Both partners touch, massage, and caress their partner's body, but they avoid any erotogenous areas; coitus and speaking are discouraged. Both partners are usually relieved when the pressure to have coitus is removed; however, if one or both are aroused, they are requested to masturbate afterwards alone. The process gradually advances to include touching around their partner's genital areas, then advances to genital touching and massage. These activities progress until coitus is permitted, but only when both are in agreement. The process takes many weeks and includes frequent homework assignments.

Sex Therapy is a specialized approach developed solely for the treatment of sexual problems while using some of the therapies already in use in the management of psychological problems. Many sexual issues can be helped by sex therapy, but many cannot; success rests on the patient's motivation, the therapist's skill, and the nature of the sexual problem. "Sex therapy is the application of professional and ethical skills to deal with the problems of sexual function of people. It assumes recognition of the concept that sexuality is of legitimate concern to professionals and that it is the right of individuals to expect knowledge when seeking remedies with sexual concerns. Sex Therapists and Clinical Psychologists focus their specialized skills to help individuals and/or couples to deal with their specific sexual concerns."[4(p1)]

Sex therapy is useful in the treatment of sexual issues related to all phases of the sexual cycle, issues of desire, arousal, and orgasm and ejaculation. Other client issues treated with sex therapy include those associated with sexual preference, gender identity, limited or relaxed sexual inhibitions, communication, chronic illness, and socially unacceptable and illegal sexual activities.

Social Skills Rehabilitation or Training includes coaching and modeling of social behaviors that are societally acceptable as well as unacceptable, and the expectation that the individual can replicate acceptable behaviors and eliminate the unacceptable social behaviors.

Start-Stop Method and the Squeeze Technique are methods used for the treatment of premature ejaculation in men, and they are reported to be effective for stopping or slowing down a potential ejaculation. The Start-Stop method requires that a man have the ability (through training) to stop stimulation of the penis midway through his excitement phase, and then allow his erection to become flaccid; he then resumes the excitement process again. This method requires self-masturbation, then masturbation by his partner, followed by gentle coitus, and finally coital thrusting if it is an appropriate time to ejaculate. The Squeeze Technique requires that a man be able to identify the period just before his ejaculation occurs, at which point he squeezes the shaft of his penis between his thumb and forefinger to stop the ejaculation; this squeeze method is often done by his partner. He allows his erection to become flaccid, and then resumes his stimulation activities until he chooses to ejaculate.

Supportive Therapy "is used primarily to reinforce a patient's ability to cope with stressors through a number of key activities, including attentively listening and encouraging expression of thoughts and feelings; assisting the individual to gain a greater understanding of their situation and alternatives; helping to buttress the individual's self-esteem and resilience; and working to instill a sense of hope. Generally, deeper examination of the individual's history and probing of underlying motivation is avoided. Supportive psychotherapy is a common form of therapy that may be provided over the short or long term, depending on the individual and the specific set of circumstances."[5 (p1)]

Surrogate Therapy is an intervention used mostly to treat sexual disorders in men, one that nowadays is both controversial and rarely recommended by sex therapists or sexologists. This approach uses the services of a sex surrogate who is paid to participate in and perform not only numerous different sex acts, but also to perform acts of day-to-day living that help clients with various perceived deficiencies. Acts that might alleviate shyness or communication problems, to rectify bad manners and mannerisms, enhance social correctness, etc. The issues are that there is money exchanged for sex, and the charge is usually expensive; consequently, sexual surrogate therapy is viewed in the same light as prostitution.

Twelve-Step Programs

"Relating to, or characteristic of a program that is designed especially to help an individual overcome an addiction, compulsion, serious shortcoming, or traumatic experience by adherence to 12 tenets emphasizing personal growth and dependence on a higher spiritual being."[6 (p1)] Use of this approach was popularized by Patrick Carnes for what he described as sex addiction. However, sex addiction is not included in the recent version of DSM-5 as a sexual diagnosis and is not accepted as a diagnosis by many clinical psychologists.

Appendix E
The Plissit Model of Sex Therapy

The PLISSIT Model was developed by Jack Annon[7] in the 1970s as a tool to improve communication between HCPs and patients with different severity levels of sexual problems. This model allows HCPs to respond to patients according to the HCP's level of theoretical and experiential sexual knowledge, clinical expertise, value system, and comfort level in discussing sexuality, and guides the HCP to refer the patient to a more appropriate provider when necessary. The model contains four levels:

Level 1: Permission Giving (P)
This level requires the HCP to provide the patient with permission to continue what he or she is doing or not continue what he or she is doing, to provide reassurance or permission; must also include the consequences to the person. There is no change in treatment. A **moderate** number of HCPs are adequately prepared to perform at this level. Referral to an expert is not usually required.

Level 2: Limited Information (LI)
This level requires the sharing of a limited amount of factual information by the HCP; for example, to discuss misconceptions, provide actual data, and dispel sexual myths. Provide simple facts only. There is no change in treatment. **Some** HCPs are adequately

prepared to perform at this level. Referral to an expert not usually required.

Level 3: Specific Suggestions (SS)
This level requires that the HCP provide specific information and the patient take specific actions; may include homework assignments. Specific suggestions must be given accurately and comfortably; if not, referral is indicated. A **few** HCPs are adequately prepared at this level. Referral to a physician, sex therapist, psychologist, or sexologist is mostly required.

Level 4: Intensive Therapy (IT)
This level occurs when the patient has sexual and/or emotional issues that are serious and guidance and management are beyond the scope of the HCP's skills and knowledge level. **Very few** HCPs are adequately prepared to perform at this level. Referral to a physician, sex therapist, psychologist, or sexologist is always required.

Appendix F

Your Attitudes Toward Unconventional Sexual Behaviors

Please Write Down Your First Thoughts

(For Your Eyes Only)

Ask yourself: What are my attitudes toward sexual behaviors that are considered unconventional by some?

Sexual Behaviors	Always Accept 5	Often Accept 4	Sometimes Accept/Reject 3	Often Reject 2	Always Reject 1
Anal sex man to woman					
Anal sex man to man					
Bestiality					
Bisexuality					
Cross dressing					
Exhibitionism					
Female to female oral sex					
Female to male oral sex					
Fetishism					
Frotteurism					
Golden showers					
Group sex					

Understanding Patients' Sexual Problems

Sexual Behaviors	Always Accepts 5	Often Accepts 4	Sometimes Accepts/Rejects 3	Often Rejects 2	Always Rejects 1
Incest					
Male to male oral sex					
Male to female oral sex					
Masturbation					
Pedophilia					
Pornography					
Prostitution					
Rape					
Sadism & Masochism					
Sexual Abuse					
Swinging					
Transvestism					
Voyeurism					

Appendix G

Supportive Interventions Guide for Children

The HCP is advised to:

1. Treat the child as an individual person not just as a child with a sexual behavior problem.
2. Exhibit a sex positive attitude during conversations and encourage the family to do the same.
3. Be the child's advocate, teacher, comforter, and provider of care within professional role.
4. Assess the child's behavior, socialization patterns, relationship with parents and with other children, toy use and active play, and language and effect.
5. Avoid letting emotions cloud objective judgment.
6. Listen actively to the child and speak truthfully; the trust of a child, if lost, is difficult to regain.
7. Engage the parents or caregivers in as many activities as possible, and keep them involved as appropriate.
8. Determine where the child is in his/her development, and

provide age-level and knowledge-level information.

9. Establish with the child his or her personal boundaries and the boundaries of others.
10. Encourage families to develop rules about sexuality, nudity, and language in the home to reduce family and child anxiety.
11. Remember that all families and all childhood upbringings are not the same.
12. Reinforce that care is primarily of the child, not of the parents.
13. Some parents may need education and perhaps psychiatric care; refer according to need.
14. Know the cultural differences that exist between the HCP, the child, and the local community.
15. Be fully cognizant of state laws regarding sexuality and children, and adhere to all mandated reporting expectations.
16. Be aware of own assumptions, fears, biases, prejudices, and existence of own stereotypical attitudes.

17. Ensure that own knowledge-base, education-base, and comfort level are more than adequate to meet the child's needs; if not, do not proceed and discuss with your administrator.
18. Be aware of and implement infection control, pain management, safety and risk management protocols within professional role (nurse, social worker, others).
19. Establish privacy rules with the child and family, and adhere to facility confidentiality and privacy protocols.

Appendix H
Supportive Interventions Guide for Adults

The HCP is advised to:

Treat the adult as an individual, not just as a person with a sexual behavior problem.

1. Exhibit a sex positive attitude during conversations and interactions.
2. Avoid heterosexist and heterocentrist attitudes in communications and interactions.
3. Be aware of own fears, biases, prejudices, sexual issues, and existence of own stereotypical attitudes.
4. Be aware of own assumptions, beliefs, values, and cultural differences that exist between the HCP and the adolescent/adult.
5. Be fully cognizant of state laws regarding sexual assault, rape, STIs, stalking, and others, and adhere to all mandated reporting expectations.
6. Ensure that HCP's knowledge-base, education-level, and comfort level are more than adequate to meet

the adolescent or adult's needs; if not, discuss with administrator.

7. Adhere to confidentiality and privacy protocols.
8. Actively listen and speak honestly, truthfully, clearly, and directly, and risk challenges and hostility.
9. Remember that sexuality and its expression are important, regardless of advancing age.
10. Be aware of the patient's diagnosis and implement plan of care according to professional role (nurse, social worker, others).
11. Use open-ended questions as much as possible.
12. Know the cultural differences that exist between the HCP, the adult/adolescent patient, and the local community.

Appendix I
How Comfortable Are You with Childhood Sexuality?
Please Write Down Your First Thoughts
(For Your Eyes Only)

1. How do you respond to the statement that children of *all* ages are sexual beings?

2. How does the perception about childhood sexuality in the United States, with its modern Western culture, differ from some other countries inside and outside of that Western culture?

3. Does seeing their parents naked or engaging in preliminary sexual activities damage young children in any way?

4. Does sleeping in the same bed with his or her parents until a child is five years old adversely affect the child?

5. What was your initial reaction when you first saw a young child masturbate? Is it the same now?

6. What actions might an adult who finds a young child masturbating take that will contribute to a child's healthy sexual outlook as an adult?

7. What actions should an adult who finds a young child masturbating *not* take?

8. Most children engage in sex-play (kissing, looking at another child's genitalia, attempting to touch another's genitalia, *playing doctor*). What is your reaction to this activity?

9. What is the worth of abstinence-only programs for children?

10. Do most children who believe they are transgender remain so as adults, or do they mostly become homosexual, bisexual, or heterosexual?

"HCPs are encouraged to face their fears about discussing patient sexuality and plunge into its daunting waters; they should lift the veil of silence, denial, and avoidance that negates the very existence of patient sexuality, and accept the fact that patients are, after all, sexual beings."

— Dr. Grace Blodgett

REFERENCES

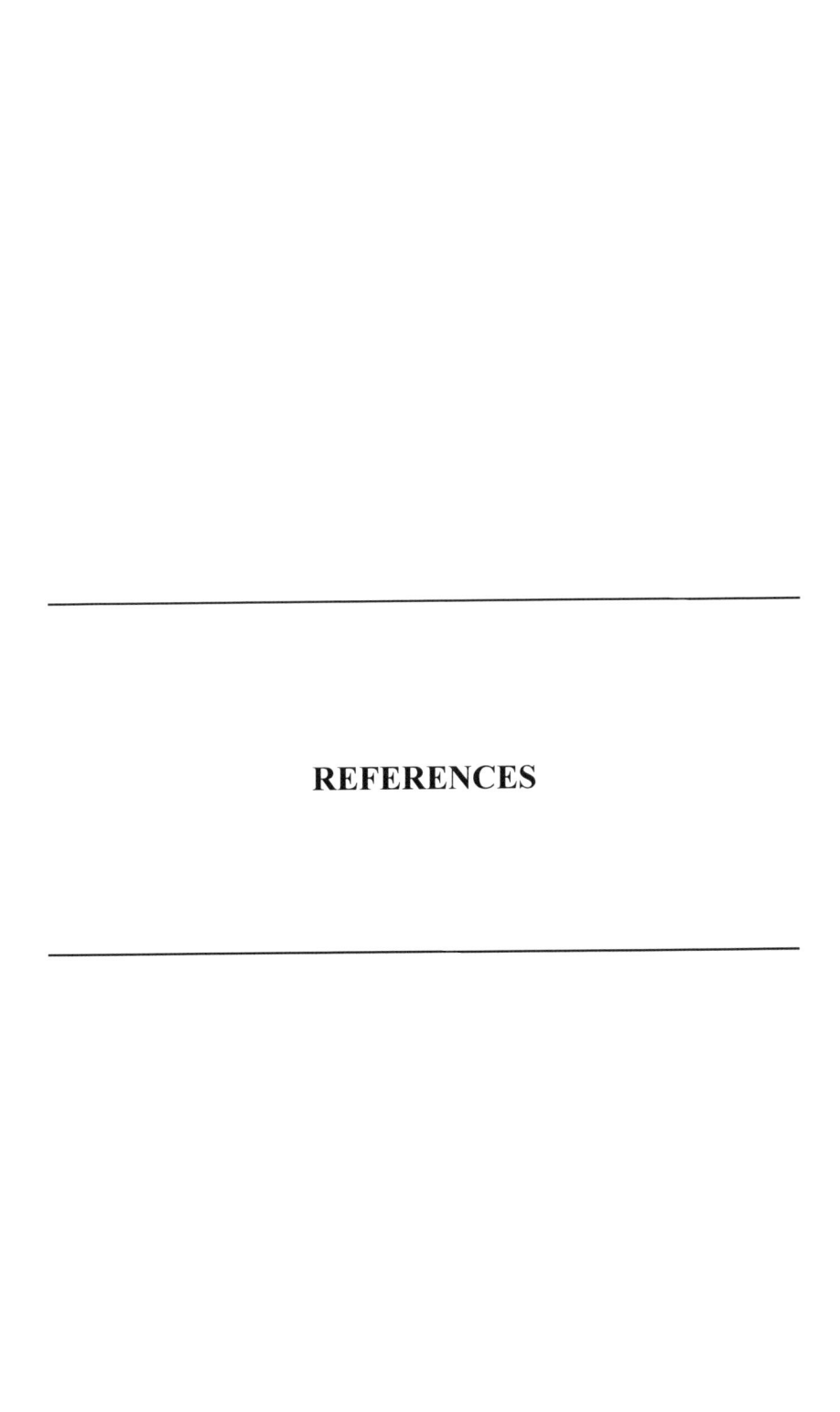

Chapter 1
Sex and Sexuality in the Healthcare Environment

1. Reynolds KE, Magnan, M. Nursing attitudes and beliefs toward human sexuality: Collaborative research promoting evidence-based practice. Journal of Advanced Nursing Practice. 2005; Sept/Oct: 19(5): 255-259. Available from: http://www.nursingcenter.com/

2. Waterhouse J. Nursing practice related to sexuality. A review and recommendations. Journal of Research Nursing. 1996 Nov: 11; 6: 412-418. Available from: http://jrn.sagepub.com/content/1/6/412.full.pdf

3. Heath H, White I. The challenge of sexuality in health care. Oxford: Blackwell Science Ltd; 2002.

4. Kalisch PA, Kalisch BJ. A comparative analysis of nurse and physician characters in the entertainment media. Journal of Advanced Nursing; 11; 1986.

5. Kelly J. Nursing's image on YouTube. American Journal of Nursing. 2012 Oct; 17. doi: 10.1097/01.NAJ.0000421012.33792.dc

6. Federation of State Medical Boards of the United States, Inc [Internet]. Addressing sexual boundaries: Guidelines for State Medical Boards. 2006. Available from: http://www.fsmb.org/Media/Default/PDF/FSMB/Advocacy/GRPOL_Sexual Boundaries.pdf

7. Haaretz Business News [Internet]. Israeli Business Poll: Half of female doctors report being sexually harassed. 2014 May 31. Available from http://www.haaretz.com/business/premium-1.534418

8. Phillips SP, Schneider MS. Sexual harassment of female doctors by patients. 1993. Available from: http://www.ncbi.nlm.nih.gov/pubmed/8247058

Chapter 2
Sexual Behaviors and Techniques According to a Person's Sexual Orientation

1. American Psychiatric Association [Internet]. Answers to your questions: For a better understanding of sexual orientation and homosexuality. Washington DC: 2006. Available from: http://www.apa.org/topics/sorientation.pdf.

Chapter 3
The Sexual Proclivities of American Adults, Societal Mores, and the Mass Media, and their Overall Impact on Sexual Behavior

1. Freud S. The interpretation of dreams. Original works published New York, NY: Avon Books; 1900. Cited by Westheimer RK, Lopater S. Human sexuality: A psychological perspective. 2nd ed. Baltimore: Lippincott Williams; 2005.

2. The Kinsey Institute. Data from Alfred Kinsey's studies. 1990. Cited by Westheimer RK, Lopater S. Human sexuality: A psychological perspective. 2nd ed. Baltimore: Lippincott Williams & Wilkins; 2005. Available from: http://www.kinseyinstitute.org/research/ak-data.html

3. Kinsey A, Pomeroy W, Martin C. Sexual behavior in the human male. 1948. Cited by Westheimer RK, Lopater S. Human sexuality: A psychological perspective. 2nded. Baltimore: Lippincott Williams & Wilkins; 2005.

4. Wikipedia [Internet]. Nocturnal emission. 2013. Available from: http://en.wikipedia.org/wiki/Nocturnal_emission

5. Leitenberg H, Henning K. Sexual fantasy. Psychology Bulletin. 2006; 117: 469-496.

6. Jones JC, Barlow DH. Self-reported frequency of sexual urges, fantasies, and masturbatory fantasies in heterosexual males and females. Archive of Sexual Behavior; 1990; 269-279. Cited by: Levay S, Valente SM. Human Sexuality. Sunderland, MA: Sinauer Associates. 2002; 216.

7. Beach F. Sexual attractivity, proceptivity, and receptivity in female mammals. Hormones and Behavior. 1976: 1(11); 105-138.

8. Fox K. Social Issues Research Centre [Internet]. SIRC guide to flirting. 2012. Available from http://www.sirc.org/publik/flirt.pdf

9. Wakin A. Huffington Post [Internet]. Cited by Sack D: Limerence and the biochemical roots of love addiction. [Place unknown]: 2012 July 5. Available from: http://www.huffingtonpost.com/david-sack-md-limerence_b_1627089.html

10. Lewis CS. A study guide of the four loves. CS Lewis Foundation [Internet]. 2001. Available from: http://www.cslewis.org/resources/studyguides/Study Guide - The Four Loves.pdf

11. Sternberg RJ. A triangular theory of love. Psychological Review. 1996: 93(2):19-135. Cited by Levay S, Valente SM. Human Sexuality. Sunderland: Sinauer Associates; 2002: 276.

12. Tennov D. Love and limerence: The experience of being in love. Briarcliff Manor: Stein & Day; 1979. Cited by Sack D. Limerence and the biochemical roots of love addiction; 2012 July 5. Available from: http://www.huffingtonpost.com/david-sack-md-limerence_b_1627089.html

13. Laumann EO, Gagnon J, Michael RT, Michaels S. The Social Organization of Sexuality: Sexual Practices in the United States. The University of Chicago Press: Chicago and London; 1994.

14. The Free Online Dictionary [Internet]. Pornography 2014. Available from http://legal-dictionary.thefreedictionary.com/pornography

15. Stanford Encyclopedia on Philosophy [Internet]. Pornography and censorship; 2012 Oct 1. Available from http://plato.stanford.edu/entries/pornography-censorship/

16. MacKinnon C. Not a moral issue. Cited by Stanford Encyclopedia of Philosophy [Internet]. Pornography and censorship. 2012 October 1. Available from http://plato.stanford.edu/entries/pornography-censorship/

17. Cooper A. Real Families, Real Answers [Internet]. [No date]. Available from: http://realfamiliesrealanswers.org/?page_id=84

18. DeAngelis T. American Psychological Association [Internet]. Monitor on Psychology. Is internet addiction real? 2000; 31: 4. Available from: http://www.apa.org/monitor/apr00/addiction.aspx

19. Ley D. et al. The emperor has no clothes: A review of the "Pornography Addiction" Model. Current sexual health reports. 2014. DOI 10.1007/s11930-014-0016-8. Cited by: Brown A. No such thing as porn "addiction" researchers say. 2014. Available from: http://link.springer.com/article/10.1007%2Fs11930-014-0016-8

20. Gallagher J. BBC News [Internet]. Scientists probe sex addict brains. 2014 July 11. Available from: http://www.bbc.com/news/health-28252612

21. American Society of Addiction Medicine. Your Brain on Porn [Internet]. Definition of addiction. 2011 Aug 15. Available from:http://yourbrainonporn.com/asam-definition-of-addiction-long-version-2011

22. Krueger R. Wikipedia [Internet]. Pornography addiction. 2014; (2). Available from http://en.wikipedia.org/wiki/Pornography_addiction

23. U.S. Legal [Internet]. Prostitution Law & Legal Definition. [No date]. Available from http://definitions.uslegal.com/p/prostitution/

24. Collins English Dictionary [Internet]. Prostitute. 2014. Available from: http://www.collinsdictionary.com/dictionary/english/prostitute?showCookiePolicy=true

25. Gilderman G. The Daily Beast [Internet]. The oldest profession-how the web transformed prostitution. 2014. Available from: http://www.dailybeast.com/articles/2012/09/10/the-oldest-profession-evolves-how-the-web-transformed-prostitution

26. Simon W, Gagnon JH. Sexual scripts: Permanence and change. Archives of Sexual Behavior. 1986 Apr 15(2): 97-120. Available from: http://www.ncbi.nlm.nih.gov/pubmed/3718206

27. Greene K, Faulkner SL. Gender, belief in the sexual double standard, and sexual talk in heterosexual dating relationships. Sex Roles. 2005 Aug 53(3/4):239-251. Available from: http://comminfo.rutgers.edu/~kgreene/research/pdf/sexroles2005.pdf

Chapter 4
Differentiating Between Expected Childhood Curiosity and Unexpected Sexual Behavior Problems of Children

1. American Psychological Association [Internet]. Washington DC: Report of the APA Task Force on the sexualization of girls; 2010. Available from; http://www.apa.org/pi/women/programs/girls/report-full.pdf

2. Nichter M. Fat talk: What girls and their parents say about dieting. Cambridge: Harvard University Press. Cited by: American Psychological Association [Internet]. Report of the APA Task Force on the Sexualization of Girls. 2010; 15. Available from: http://www.apa.org/pi/women/programs/girls/report-full.pdf

3. Zucker KJ. "On the natural history" of gender identity in children. Journal of the American Academy of Childhood Adolescence Psychiatry. 2008; 47:1361-1363. Cited by: Byne W, Bradley, S, Coleman, E, Eyler, E, Green, R, Menvielle, E, Meyer-Bahlberg, H, Pleak, R, Tompkins. Report of the American Psychiatric Association Task Force on Treatment of Gender Identity Disorder. Archive of Sexual Behavior. 2012 Aug 41(4):759-96. Available from: http://www.ncbi.nlm.nih.gov/pubmed/22736225

4. DSM-5. American Psychiatric Association [Internet]. Gender dysphoria; 2013; Available from: http://www.dsm5.org/Documents/Gender%20Dysphoria%20Fact%20Sheet.pdf

5. WebMD [Internet]. When you don't feel at home with your gender. 2014 Sept 24. Available from: http://www.webmd.com/sex/gender-identity-disorder

6. Spiegel A. Gender identity disorder in children. Wikipedia [Internet]. Gender identity disorder in children; 2008 May 7. Two families grapple with sons' gender differences: psychologists take two different approaches in therapy. National Public Radio. Available from: http://en.m.wikipedia.org/wiki/Gender_identity_disorder_in_children

7. Wallien MS, Cohen-Kettenis PT. Psych-social outcomes of gender-dysphoric children. Journal of the Academy of Child and Adolescent Psychiatry. 2008 Dec; 47(12):1413-1423. Available from: http://www.ncbi.nlm.nih.gov/pubmed/18981931

8. Diamond M. Pacific Center for Sex and Society. University of Hawaii. Medical change. Milton Diamond challenges gender assignment. Available from: www.hawaii.edu/PCSS/biblio/articles/2000to2004/2002-medical-change.html

9. Turner's Syndrome Society of the United States [Internet]. Turner's syndrome fact sheet; 2013. Available from: http://www.turnersyndrome.org/ - fact-or-myth/c1bqb9

10. Klinefelter Syndrome-XXY. James Madison University; 2014; Available from: http://www.psyc.jmu.edu/school/documents/Klinefelter.pdf

11. WebMD [Internet]. Men's Health: XYY syndrome; 2014 Sept 04. Available from: http://www.webmd.com/men/xyy-syndrome

12. Genetics Home Reference [Internet]. 47,XYY Syndrome; 2009 Jan. Available from: http://www.ghr.nlm.nih.gov/condition/47xyy-syndrome

13. Otter M, TRM Schrander-Stumpel C, Curfs LMG. Triple X syndrome: a review of the literature. European Journal of Human Genetics; 2010 Mar; 18(3): 265-271. Available from: http://www.ncbi.nlm.nih.gov/pmc/articles/PMC2987225/

14. Medline Plus [Internet]. National Institute of Health. Androgen insensitivity syndrome; 2012 July 19. Available from: http://www.nlm.nih.gov/medlineplus/ency/article/001180.htm

15. Urology Care Foundation [Internet]. Hypospadias; 2013 Mar. Available from: http://www.urologyhealth.org/urology/index.cfm?article=130

16. Mayo Clinic [Internet]. Undescended testicle; 2013; Available from: http://www.mayoclinic.org/diseases-conditions/.../con-20037877

17. Agency for Healthcare Research and Quality [Internet]. Evaluation and treatment of cryptorchidism; 2012 Dec 11. Available from: http://effectivehealthcare.ahrq.gov/index.cfm/search-for-guides-reviews-and-reports/?productid=1352&pageaction=displayproduct

18. Merke DP. Approach to the adult with congenital adrenal hyperplasia due to 21 hydroxylase deficiency. 2008 Mar. Cited by Wilson TA: Congenital Adrenal Hyperplasia. 2012. Available from Medscape: http://emedicine.medscape.com/article/919218-overview

19. MedlinePlus [Internet]. Congenital adrenal hyperplasia; 2014 Feb 3. Available from: http://www.nlm.nih.gov/medlineplus/ency/article/000411.htm

20. Speiser PW. Congenital adrenal hyperplasia owing to 21-hydroxylase deficiency. Endocrinology Metabolism Clinics of North America. 2001 Mar 30:31-59. Available from: http://www.ncbi.nlm.nih.gov/pubmed/?term=11344938

21. U.S. National Library of Medicine [Internet]. PubMed Health. Congenital adrenal hyperplasia; 2014 Feb 3. Available from: http://www.ncbi.nlm.nih.gov/pubmedhealth/PMH0001448/

22. Androgen Excess Society [Internet]. Congenital Adrenal Hyperplasia (CAH); 2012. Available from: http://www.ae-society.org/Congenital_Adrenal_Hyperplasia

23. Beh HG, Diamond M. David Reimer's legacy: Limiting parental discretion. Cardozo Journal of Law and Gender. 2006: 125(1):5-30. Available from: http://www.hawaii.edu/PCSS/biblio/articles/2005to2009/2006-david-reimers-legacy.html

24. Whiteaker D. What every nurse needs to know about the clinical aspects of child abuse. American Nurse Today. 2010 July: 5(7). Available from: http://www.americannursetoday.com/what-every-nurse-needs-to-know-about-the-clinical-aspects-of-child-abuse/

25. Child Welfare Information Gateway [Internet]. Child sexual abuse; 2008. Available from: https://www.childwelfare.gov/pubs/usermanuals/sexabuse/sexabusef.cfm

26. American Psychological Association: Sexual abuse [Internet]; 2013. Available from: http://www.apa.org/pubs/info/brochures

27. Stavrianopoulos T, Gourvelou O. The role of the nurse in child sex abuse in the USA. Human Science Journal. 2012 Oct-Dec: 6(4):647- 653.

28. World Health Organization. The World Health Report. 2002. Cited by: Johnson RJ. Advances in understanding and treating childhood sexual abuse: Implications for research and policy. 2008 Jan-Mar: 31(1): s24-s31. Available from: http://www.nursingcenter.com/lnc/JournalArticle?Article_ID=763931

29. Laumann EO, Gagnon J, Michael RT, Michaels S. The Social Organization of Sexuality: Sexual Practices in the United States. Chicago and London: University of Chicago Press; 1994.

30. Brown A, Finkelhorn D. Impact of child sexual abuse: a review of the research. Psychological Bulletin. 1986 99(1): 66-77. Available from: http://psycnet.apa.org/index.cfm?fa=buy.optionToBuy&id=1986-14683-001

31. Office of Juvenile Justice and Delinquency Prevention [Internet]. Recognizing when a child's injury or illness is caused by abuse. U.S. Department of Justice; 2004 July: 647-653 Available from: http://www.ojjdp.gov/pubs/243908.pdf

32. Giardino AP, Finkel MA. Evaluation of child sex abuse. Pediatric Annals. 2005; 34: 382-394.

33. The California Evidence-Based Clearinghouse for Child Welfare. Sexual behavior problems in children, treatment of. 2014. Available from: http://www.cebc4cw.org/topic/sexual-behavior-problems-in-children-treatment-of

34. Rich P. Understanding, assessing and rehabilitating juvenile sex offenders. 2nd Edition New York: Wiley; 2011. Cited by NSPCC [Internet]. Harmful sexual behavior. NSPCC research briefing. 2013 July 1. Available from: http://www.nspcc.org.uk/globalassets/documents/information-service/research-briefing-child-sexual-abuse.pdf

35. Bonner B, Walker CE, Berliner L. Children with sexual behavior problems: Assessment and treatment. Final Report, Grant no 90-CA-1469. National Center on Child Abuse and Neglect. Administration for Child, Youth, and Families. U.S. Department of Health and Human services; 1991. Available from: http://www.dshs.wa.gov/pdf/ca/CSBPReport.pdf

36. Kellogg ND. Clinical Report—The evaluation of sexual behaviors in children. American Academy of Pediatrics. 2009 September: 124(3): 992-998. Available from: http://pediatrics.aappublications.org/content/124/3/992.short

37. Chaffin M, Berliner L, Block R, Cavanaugh-Johnson T et al. Association for the Treatment of Sexual Abusers. Child maltreatment. 2008 May;13(2):199-218.

38. Smallbone S, Marshall W, Wortley R. Preventing child sexual abuse: evidence, policy and practice. Devon: Willan Publishing; 2009. Cited by NSPCC [Internet]. Harmful sexual behavior. NSPCC research briefing; 2013 July: 1. Available from: http://www.nspcc.org.uk/globalassets/documents/information-service/research-briefing-child-sexual-abuse.pdf

REFERENCES

39. World Health Organization [Internet]. Female genital mutilation; 2014 Feb. Available from: http://www.who.int/mediacentre/factsheets/fs241/en/

40. UNFPA [Internet]. Genital mutilation/cutting: Promoting gender equality; 2014. Available from: http://www.unfpa.org/gender/practices2.htm

41. Johansen REB, Nafissatou JD, Laverack G, Leye E. What works and what does not: A discussion of popular approaches for the abandonment of FGM. Obstetrics and Gynecology International. 2012. Available from: http://www.hindawi.com/journals/ogi/2013/348248/

42. Wild Iris Medical Education [Internet]. Sexually transmitted diseases (STDs); 2012. Available from: http://www.wildirismedicaleducation.com/courses/402/index_nceu.html

43. Centers for Disease Control and Prevention. Morbidity and Mortality Report. STDs treatment guidelines. 2010 Dec 17: 59(RR12); 1-110. Available from: http://www.cdc.gov/mmwr/preview/mmwrhtml/rr5912a1.htm

44. Botash AS. SUNY Upstate Medical University. Appendix A: Post assault testing and therapy; 2014. Available from: http://www.childabusemd.com/appendices/appendix-A.shtml

Chapter 5
High-Risk Sexual Behaviors By and Against Adolescents, and the Challenges They Present

1. Stuckman-Johnson A. Tactics of sexual coercion. When men and women won't take no for an answer. Florida Department of Health. 2002. Cited by McKoy MS, Oelschlanger J. Sexual Coercion Awareness and Prevention. Florida Institute of Technology. [No date]. Available from: http://www.fit.edu/caps/documents/SexualCoercion_000.pdf

2. Vedantam S. What does sexual coercion say about a society? National Public Radio [Internet]; 2013 May. Available from: http://www.npr.org/2013/05/10/182654664/what-does-sexual-coercion-say-about-a-society/

3. The American College of Obstetricians and Gynecologists [Internet]. Adolescent Facts. Pregnancy, births and STDs; 2009. Available from: http://www.acog.org/-/media/Department-Publications/AdolescentFactsPregnancyAndSTDs.pdf?dmc=1&ts=20141113T1348132624

4. Ventura SJ, Abma JC, Mosher WD, Henshaw SK. Estimated pregnancy rates by outcome in the United States 1990-2004. National Vital Statistics Report. 2008; 56(15): 1-25, 28. Cited by: The American College of Obstetricians and Gynecologists [Internet]. Adolescent Facts. Pregnancy, births and STDs; 2002; Available from: http://www.acog.org/-/media/Department-Publications/AdolescentFactsPregnancyAndSTDs.pdf?dmc=1&ts=20141113T1351004190

5. Martin JA, Hamilton BE, Sutton PD, Ventura SJ, Menacker F, Kirmeyer S et al. Births: final data for 2006. National Vital Statistics Report. 2007; 57(7): 1-102. Available from: http://www.cdc.gov/nchs/data/nvsr/nvsr57/nvsr57_07.pdf. Cited by: The American College of Obstetricians and Gynecologists [Internet]. Adolescent Facts. Pregnancy, births and STDs; 2009. Available from: http://www.acog.org/-/media/Department-Publications/AdolescentFactsPregnancyAndSTDs.pdf?dmc=1&ts=20141113T1351004190

6. Eaton DK, Kann L, Kinchner S, Shanklin S, Ross J, Hawkins J. et al. Youth risk behavior surveillance—United States 2007. Center for Disease Control and Prevention. MMWR Surveill Summ. 2008; 57(SS-4): 1-131. Cited by: The American College of Obstetricians and Gynecologists [Internet]. Adolescent Facts. Pregnancy, births and STDs; 2009. Available from: http://www.acog.org/-/media/Department-Publications/AdolescentFactsPregnancyAndSTDs.pdf?dmc=1&ts=20141113T1351004190

7. The Guttmacher Institute [Internet]. Teen pregnancy: Trends and lessons learned; 2002 Feb: 5(1). Available from: http://www.guttmacher.org/pubs/tgr/05/1/gr050107.html

8. Daroch J, Singh S, Frost J, and the Study Team. Differences in teenage pregnancy rates among five developed countries. The roles of sexual activity and contraceptive use. Family Planning Perspectives. 2001; 33(6). Available from: http://www.guttmacher.org/pubs/journals/3324401.html

9. Centers for Disease Control [Internet]. Youth risk behaviors

surveillance—United States 2011. MMWR; 2012: 61(SS-4). Cited by: Centers for Disease Control [Internet]. Sexual risk behavior: HIV, STD, & Teen pregnancy prevention; 2004 Jun. Available from: http://www.cdc.gov/healthyyouth/sexualbehaviors/index.htm

10. National Library of Medicine [Internet]. Adolescent pregnancy; 2011. Available from: http://www.nlm.nih.gov/medlineplus/ency/article/001516.htm

11. Centers for Disease Control [Internet]. Sexual risk behavior: HIV, STD, & Teen pregnancy prevention; 2004 Jun. Available from: http://www.cdc.gov/HealthyYouth/sexualbehaviors/

12. Boston Public Health Commission [Internet]. Fact sheet: intimate partner violence and teen dating violence; 2014. Available from: http://www.bphc.org/whatwedo/violence-prevention/start-strong/Documents/Intimate_Teen_Dating.pdf - search=intimate partner violence

13. Mayo Clinic [Internet]. Signs and symptoms of frequently occurring STDs; 2013 July. Available from: http://www.mayoclinic.org/diseases-conditions/sexually-transmitted-diseases-stds/basics/symptoms/con-20034128

14. Family Planning Council [Internet]. Family planning council: STD Facts. [No date]. Available from: http://www.familyplanning.org/reprofacts_stds.shtml

15. Centers for Disease Control [Internet]. CDC fact sheet. Incidence, prevalence, and cost of sexually transmitted

diseases in the United States; 2013 Feb. Available from: http://www.cdc.gov/std/stats/STI-Estimates-Fact-Sheet-Feb-2013.pdf

16. National Library of Medicine [Internet]. MedlinePlus. Reportable diseases summary; 2013 May. Available from: http://www.nlm.nih.gov/medlineplus/ency/article/001929.htm

17. Centers for Disease Control [Internet] Morbidity and Mortality Weekly Guidelines. Sexually transmitted diseases treatment; 2010. Available from: http://www.cdc.gov/mmwr/preview/mmwrhtml/rr5912a1.htm

18. The Free Dictionary [Internet]. Rape; 2014. Available from: http://www.thefreeedictionary.com/rape

19. Rape, Abuse, & Incest National Network [Internet]. Acquaintance Rape; 2009. Available from: https://www.rainn.org/get-information/types-of-sexual-assault/acquaintance-rape

20. Fisher BS, Cullen FT, Turner MG. The sexual victimization of college women. Bureau of Justice. Bureau Justice Statistics; 2000. Available from: https://www.ncjrs.gov/pdffiles1/nij/182369.pdf

21. Groth N. Men who rape: The psychology of the offender. New York: Plenus Press; 1979; 44-45; 1. ISBN 0-306-40268-8. Cited by: Wikipedia [Internet]. Types of rape; 2013 Aug. Available from: http://www.en.wikipedia.org/wiki/Types_of_rape

22. Humphrey S, Kahn A. The problem of acquaintance rape of college students; 2000. Cited by: Sampson R. Acquaintance rape of college students. Guide No 17. University of Albany, 2002; Available from: http://www.popcenter.org/problems/rape/print

Chapter 6
Problems That People Who Are Gay, Lesbian, or Bi-Sexual Experience as a Result of Their Sexual Orientation

1. American Psychological Association [Internet]. Definitions of terms—sex, gender, gender identity, sexual orientation; 2011. Available from http://www.apa.org/pi/lgbt/

2. DeAngelis T. New data on lesbian, gay and bisexual mental health. New findings overturn previous beliefs. American Psychological Association. 2002 Feb: 33(2). Available from: http://www.apa.org/monitor/feb02/newdata.aspx

3. Shankle MD. The handbook of lesbian, gay, bisexual, and transgender public health: A practitioner's guide to service. New York: Haworth Press; 2006: 39.

4. Marazzo JM, Koutsky LA, Hansfield HH. Sexually transmitted disease clients who report same-sex behavior. International Journal of STD and AIDS, 12(1), 41-46. Cited by: Shankle MD. The handbook of lesbian, gay, bisexual, and transgender public health: A practitioner's guide to service. New York: Haworth Press; 2006: 90.

5. Royal College of Psychiatrists [Internet]. A submission to the Church of England's listening exercise on human sexuality. Environment and sexual orientation; 2007: 6. Available from: http://www.rcpsych.ac.uk/workinpsychiatry/specialinterestgroups/gaylesbian/submissiontothecofe.aspx. Cited by: Wikipedia [Internet]. Retrieved 2013 June

13. Available from: http://www.en.wikipedia.org/wiki/environment_and_sexual_orientation

6. American Psychological Association [Internet]. Answers to your questions: for a better understanding of sexual orientation and homosexuality; 2008: 6. Available from: http://www.apa.org/topics/lgbt/orientation.pdf

7. Laumann E, Gagnon JH, Michael RT, Michaels S. National Health and Social Life Study. The social organization of sexuality: Sexual practices in the United States. Chicago: University of Chicago Press; 1994. Cited by: The Kinsey Institute. Prevalence of homosexuality. Brief summary of U.S. Studies 2014: 3. Available from: http://www.kinseyinstitute.org/resources/bib-homoprev.html

8. Herek G. Facts about homosexuality and child molestation 1997-2013; BLOG [Internet]. Available from:
9. http://psychology.ucdavis.edu/faculty_sites/rainbow/html/facts_molestation.html

10. Jenny et al. Are children at risk for sexual abuse by homosexuals? Pediatrics; 94; 41-44. Cited by: Herek G. Facts about homosexuality and child molestation. 1997-2013; BLOG [Internet]: Available from: http://psychology.ucdavis.edu/faculty_sites/rainbow/html/facts_molestation.html

11. American Institute of Bisexuality [Internet]. The Klein sexual orientation grid. Routledge: Taylor and Francis; 2012. Available from: http://www.americaninstituteofbisexuality.org/thekleingrid/

12. Kinsey A, Pomeroy W, Martin C. Kinsey sexual orientation grid. Sexual behavior in the human male. Philadelphia: W.B Saunders; 1948.

13. Jones JM. Most in U.S. say gay and lesbian bias is a serious problem. Gallup poll [Internet]. USA.Today; 2012 Dec 6. Available from: http://www.gallup.com/poll/159113/most-say-gay-lesbian-bias-serious-problem.aspx

14. Gay Marriage ProCon [Internet]. 33 states have legal same-sex marriage, 17 still have same-sex marriage bans; 2014 Nov 13. Available from: http://gaymarriage.procon.org/view.resource.php?resourceID=004857

Chapter 7
The Sexual and Social Problems Individuals with Gender Dysphoria Encounter

1. Mayer KH, Bradford JB, Mackadon HJ, Stall R, Goldhammer H, Landers S. Sexual and gender minority health: what we know and what needs to be done. American Journal of Public Health. 2008 Jun; 98(6): 989-995. Available from: http://www.lmunet.edu/dcom/hec/PDFs/Sexual%20and%20Gender%20Minority%20Health.pdf

2. American Psychiatric Association. Diagnostic and Statistical Manual of Mental Disorder. DSM-5. Washington DC: APA; 2013.

3. De Vries LC, Cohen-Kettenis PT, Delemarre-van der Waal H. Caring for transgender adolescents in BC: Suggested guidelines. Vancouver Coastal Health, Transcend, Transgender Support and Education Society, and the Canadian Rainbow Health Coalition. 2006; A2. Available from: http://www.amsa.org/AMSA/Libraries/Committee_Docs/CaringForTransgenderAdolescents.sflb.ashx

4. Healthy People 2020 [Internet]. Transgender health fact sheet; 2010 Nov. Available from: http://www.lgbttobacco.org/files/TransgenderHealthFact.pdf

5. Transgender Law [Internet]. Transgender Issues: Fact Sheet. [No date]. Available from: http://www.transgenderlaw.org/resources/transfactsheet.pdf

6. Feldman JI, Goldberg J. Transgender primary medical care. New York: Haworth Press; 2006.

7. Wallien MS, Cohen-Kettenis PT. Psychosexual outcome of gender-dysphoric children. Journal of the American Academy of Child and Adolescent Psychiatry. 2008 Dec; 47(12):1413-23. Available from: http://www.ncbi.nlm.nih.gov/pubmed/18981931

Chapter 8
Sexual Dysfunctions in Men and Women and Their Contributing Learned Behaviors

1. Laumann EO, Gagnon J, Michael RT, Michaels S. The Social Organization of Sexuality. Sexual Practices in the United States. The University of Chicago Press: Chicago and London; 1994.

2. Basson R, Leiblum S, Brotto L, et al. Definitions of women's sexual dysfunction reconsidered: advocating expansion and revision. Journal of Psychosomatic Obstetrical Gynecology. 2003 24(4):221-229.

3. Mayo Clinic [Internet]. Erectile dysfunction; 2012 Feb 10. Available from: http://www.mayoclinic.org/diseases-conditions/erectile-dysfunction/basics/definition/con-20034244?_ga=1.252450441.1059761743.1415908881

4. Wikipedia [Internet]. Anorgasmia; 2014 Aug 5: Available from: http://www.en.wikipedia.org/wiki/anorgasmia

5. American Urological Association [Internet]. Premature ejaculation; 2013. Available from https://www.auanet.org/education/guidelines/premature-ejaculation.cfm

6. Advanced Urological Care [Internet]. Ejaculation Dysfunction Treatment-Anejaculation; 2014. Available from: http://www.urologicalcare.com/ejaculation-dysfunction/anejaculation/

7. WebMD [Internet]. Retrograde ejaculation; 2014. Available from:

http://www.webmd.com/sexual-conditions/retrograde-ejaculation

8. Petersen CD, Lundvall L, Kristensen E, Giraldi A. Vulvodynia. Definition, diagnosis, and treatment. Acta Obste Gynecol Scand. 2008: 87(9):893-90. Cited by Ventolini G. Measuring treatment outcomes in women with vulvodynia. Journal of Clinical Medical Research. 2011 Mar. Available from: http://www.ncbi.nlm.nih.gov/pmc/articles/PMC3140924/

9. National Vulvodynia Association [Internet]; 2013. Available from: https://www.nva.org/

10. Vaginismus Official Site [Internet]; 2014. What is vaginismus? Available from: https://www.vaginismus.com/faqs/vaginismus-questions/what-is-vaginismus

11. Mayo Clinic [Internet]; 2012 Jan. Painful intercourse (dyspareunia). Available from: http://www.mayoclinic.org/diseases-conditions/painful-intercourse/basics/definition/con-20033293

12. Wadsworth Family Medicine [Internet]. Dyspareunia; 2013. Available from: http://www.wadsworthfamilymedicine.com/pdfs/Women/Handouts/Dyspareunia.pdf

13. Choices in Health [Internet]. Dyspareunia (painful intercourse); 2013. Available from: http://www.choicespc.net/dyspareunia

14. Barnas J, Parker M, Guhring P, Mulhall JP. The utility of tamsulosin in the management of orgasm-associated pain. A pilot analysis. European Urology. 2005 Mar: 47(3):365. Available from: http://www.ncbi.nlm.nih.gov/pubmed/15716202

Chapter 9
Sexuality Concerns in Adults with a Chronic Illness, a Severe Disability, an End-Of-Life Illness or Older Age

1. Alzheimer's Society, UK [Internet]. Sex and Dementia; 2012. Available from: http://www.alzheimers.org.uk/site/scripts/documents_info.php?documentID=129

2. Alzheimer's Foundation of America [Internet]. About Alzheimer's; 2014 Jun 5. Available from: http://www.alzfdn.org/AboutAlzheimers/definition.html

3. Macmillan Cancer Support. Sexuality and Cancer. London: Macmillan Cancer Support. 2012; 15-16.

4. Berger AM, Abernathy AP, Atkinson E et al. Cancer-related fatigue. Journal National Cancer Network. 2010: 8(8):904-930. Cited by: Keeney CE, Head BA. Palliative nursing care of the patient with cancer-related fatigue. Journal Hospital and Palliative Nursing. 2011; 13(5):270-278. Available from: http://www.medscape.com/viewarticle/750313

5. National Diabetes Clearing House [Internet]. Causes of diabetes; 2011. Available from: http://diabetes.niddk.nih.gov/dm/pubs/causes/index.aspx

6. National Diabetes Clearing House [Internet]. Sexual and urologic problems of diabetes; 2011. Available from: http://diabetes.niddk.nih.gov/dm/pubs/sup/

7. De Bernardi G, Franciosi M, Belfiglio M, Di Nardo B. et al.

Erectile dysfunctions and quality of life in Type 2 diabetic patients. Diabetes Care. 2002 Feb; 25(2):284-291. Available from: http://care.diabetesjournals.org/content/25/2/284.full

8. National Multiple Sclerosis Society [Internet]. Definition of MS; 2014. Available from: http://www.nationalmssociety.org/What-is-MS/Definition-of-MS

9. National Multiple Sclerosis Society [Internet]. Who gets MS? [No date]. Available from: http://www.nationalmssociety.org/What-is-MS/Who-Gets-MS

10. AAIDD [Internet]. Frequently asked questions on intellectual disability; 2013. Available from: http://aaidd.org/intellectual-disability/definition/faqs-on-intellectual-disability

11. Disabled World [Internet]. Disability sexual information on sex and sexual issues with disabilities; [No date]. Available from: http://www.disabled-world.com/disability/sexuality/

12. National Disability Authority [Internet]. A strategy for equality, sexuality and relationships; 2007. Available from: http://nda.ie/Disability-overview/Key-Policy-Documents/Sectoral-plans/A-Strategy-for-Equality.html

13. Sexuality and Disability [Internet]. Mythbusting; [No date]. Available from: http://www.sexualityanddisability.org/sexuality/mythbusting.aspx

14. Irwin M. Sexuality and people with disabilities. Indiana Institute on Disability and Community [Internet]; 2012. Available from: http://www.iidc.indiana.edu/?pageId=2502

15. European Association for Palliative Care. Sexuality in palliative care. 2004 Oct. Cited by Palliative Medicine. 18(7); 630 – 637. Available from: http://pmj.sagepub.com/content/18/7/630.abstract

16. Arensmeyer K. Nursing management of patients with cancer-related anorexia. 2012. Available from: http://www.oncolink.org/resources/article.cfm?id=1006

Chapter 10
High Sexual Desire Disorders and Sexual Compulsivity in Men and Women, and the Learned Behaviors that Contribute to Their Sexually Compulsive Actions

1. Kafka MP. Therapy for sexual impulsivity: the paraphilias and paraphilia-related disorders. Psychiatric Times [Internet]; 1996 Jun 1. Available from: http://www.psychiatrictimes.com/articles/therapy-sexual-impulsivity-paraphilias-and-paraphilia-related-disorders

2. Brain Physics [Internet]. Sexual compulsivity and sexual addiction. Defining paraphilias and related disorders; 2014. Available from: http://www.brainphysics.com/paraphilias.php

3. McManus M, Hargreaves P, Rainbow L, Allison L. Paraphilias: definition, diagnosis and treatment. F1000Prime Rep. 2013; 5:36. Available from: http://www.ncbi.nlm.nih.gov/pmc/articles/PMC3769077/

Chapter 11
A General Overview of Paraphilias and Paraphilic Disorders. Eight DSM-5 Selected Paraphilias and Paraphilic Disorders, DSM-5 Specified and Unspecified Paraphilias and Paraphilic Disorders, and Examples of Non-DSM-5 Paraphilic Disorders

1. American Psychiatric Association. Diagnostic and Statistical Manual of Mental Disorders. 5th ed. American Psychiatric Association. Washington, DC: 2013:685-705.

2. American Psychiatric Association [Internet]. Paraphilic Disorders Fact Sheet-DSM-5; 2013. Available from: http://www.dsm5.org/Documents/Paraphilic%20Disorders%20Fact%20Sheet.pdf

3. Brannon GE, Bienenfeld D, Levay R, Memon MA, Talavera F. Paraphilic disorders. Medscape [Internet]; [No date]. Available from: http://emedicine.medscape.com/article/291419-overview

4. Kafka M. Therapy for sexual impulsivity: The paraphilias and paraphilia-related disorders. Psychiatric Times [Internet]; 1996 Jun 1. Available from: http://www.psychiatrictimes.com/articles/therapy-sexual-impulsivity-paraphilias-and-paraphilia-related-disorders

5. Freund K, Watson R. Mapping the boundaries of courtship disorders. Journal of Sex Research. 1990 Nov; 27(4):589-606. Available from: http://robinjwilson.com/articles/Freund-Watson_Mapping.pdf

6. Money J. Lovemaps: A theory for the paraphilias. New York, Irvington Publishers. 1996.

7. Frey R. Exhibitionism. Encyclopedia of Mental Disorders [Internet]; 2002. Available from: http://www.Minddisorders.com/Del-Fi/Exhibitionism.html

8. Kaplan MS, Krueger RB. Cognitive-behavioral treatment of the paraphilias. Israel Journal of Psychiatry Related Science. 2012; 49(40);291-6. Available from: http://www.ncbi.nlm.nih.gov/pubmed/23585466

9. Bradford JMW, McDonald W. The treatment of sexual deviation using a pharmacological approach. Journal of Sex Research. 2000 Aug; 37(3):248-257. Available from: http://www.tandfonline.com/doi/abs/10.1080/00224490009552045#.VGUhiVMeIYB

10. Psychiatry Online [Internet]. Diagnostic and Statistical Manual of Mental Disorders. 5th ed. Paraphilic disorders; [No date]. Available from: http://dsm.psychiatryonline.org/doi/book/10.1176/appi.books.9780890425596

11. Marvin R. Proposed DSM-5 revisions to sexual and gender identity disorder criteria. Virtual Mentor [Internet]. 2010 Aug; 8:673-677. Available from: http://virtualmentor.ama-assn.org/2010/08/msoc1-1008.html

12. American Psychiatric Association. Diagnostic and Statistical Manual of Mental Disorders. Test Revision. DSM-IV-R. 4th ed. American Psychiatric Association. Washington, DC: 2000

13. Kafka M. The DSM diagnostic criteria for fetishism. Archives of Sexual Behavior. 2010; 39; 357-362. Available from: http://drmarkgriffiths.wordpress.com/2012/03/13/perverse-curse-or-worse-survival-of-the-fetish/

14. Abel CG, Osborne VA. The paraphilias. The extent and nature of sexually deviant and criminal behavior. Psychiatric Clinics of America. 15: 675-687.

15. Darcangelo S. Fetishism: Psychopathology and theory. In Sexual Deviance, Second Edition: Theory, Assessment, and Treatment. New York: Guilford Press; 2008.

16. Lanning KV. Child molesters: A behavioral analysis. 4th ed. Alexandria: National Center for Exploited Children; 2001. Cited by: Hall RCW. A profile of pedophiles, characteristics of offenders, recidivism, treatment outcomes, and forensic issues. Available from: http://www.ncbi.nlm.nih.gov/pubmed/17418075

17. Dickey R, Nussbaum D, Chevolleau K, Davidson H. Age as a differential characteristic of rapists, pedophiles, and sexual sadists. Journal of Sex Marital Therapy. 2002; 28; 211-21.

18. Journal of Sex Marital Therapy. Age as a differential characteristic of rapists, pedophiles, and sexual sadists. 2002; 28; 211-21.

19. Encyclopedia of Mental Disorders [Internet]. Sexual masochism; [No date]. Available from: http://www.minddisorders.com/Py-Z/Sexual-masochism.html

20. Collective Social Services [Internet]. Sexual sadism; 2010. Available from: http://www.regionalcenter.org/mental-heath/sexual-sadism

21. Encyclopedia of Mental Disorders [Internet]. Voyeurism; [No date]. Available from: http://www.minddisorders.com/Py-Z/Voyeurism.html

Appendices

1. Foley S, Kope S, Sugrue DP. Sex matters for women. New York: The Guildford Press: 2002. Available from: http://www.amazon.com/Sex-Matters-Women-Complete-Taking/dp/1572307005

2. Priority Health [Internet]. 5 Ps of Taking a Sexual History. Adapted from sexually transmitted diseases and treatment guidelines. Center for Disease Control. 2006 Sept. Available from: https://www.priorityhealth.com/provider/clinical-resources/~/media/documents/preventive-care/chlamydia/five-ps-taking-sexual-history-checklist.pdf

3. Interpersonal Society for Interpersonal Psychotherapy [Internet]. About IPT; 2014. Available from: http://interpersonalpsychotherapy.org/about-ipt/

4. American Board of Sexology [Internet]. What is sex therapy? [No date]. Available from: http:www.americanboardofsexology.com/whatis.htm

5. University of Toronto [Internet]. Supportive psychotherapy. Toronto: Counseling and Psychological Services; [No date]. Available from: www.caps.utoronto.ca/Services-Offered/Individual-Psychotherapy/Supportive-psychotherapy.htm

6. Merriam-Webster Medical Dictionary [Internet]. 12 step medical definition; [No date]. Available from: www.merriam-webster.com/medical/12-step

7. Annon J. Behavioral treatment of sexual problems: brief therapy. New York: Harper and Row Medical Department; 1976.

ABOUT DR. GRACIE

Dr. Gracie grew up in the outskirts of London, England, and from 1959 to 1962 attended nursing school at The Royal London Hospital (of Jack the Ripper and Elephant Man fame) in the East End of London. She emigrated to the U.S. the end of 1967 with her former husband, Joe, and her two sons, Mark and Paul.

She married her husband of 40 years, Peter, in 1975, and with the two boys they moved to Salt Lake City, Utah, where they lived and worked for 17 years. Dr. Gracie and Peter had two more children, Kate and Jonathan, and are now the very proud grandparents of six wonderful granddaughters: Gillian, Avery, Maysea, India, Isabelle, and Lilly. They had the opportunity to move to beautiful Kaneohe, Hawaii, and exchanged the snowy winters for year-round sun and sea. After 22 years of living in Hawaii, they do not regret their decision, and they look forward to remaining in Hawaii for a wonderful retirement.

Dr. Gracie is a seasoned healthcare professional, with over 50 years' experience in the field of applied nursing and nursing education, combined with over 20 years' experience in the discipline of human sexuality. Her time in the healthcare world spans from 1959 as a 19-year-old probationary nurse to the present, during which time her chosen profession has served her extremely well.

Dr. Gracie obtained her registered nurse status in England in 1962, and her midwifery certification in 1966. When she first arrived in the U.S. in 1967, she worked as a staff nurse at Columbia Presbyterian Hospital, until she was promoted to a head nurse position there a few years later. She became a nurse educator and then medical/surgical nursing director at Roosevelt Hospital where she remained until their family moved to Salt Lake City in 1975.

After their move to Salt Lake City and over the next 15 years, Dr. Gracie was a staff nurse, a head nurse, and then director of nursing for medical services and post-intensive care services at Holy Cross Hospital. She then developed a successful consultation business to prepare general and rehabilitation hospitals for review by Joint Commission evaluators.

Dr. Gracie opened the University of Phoenix, Hawaii Campus, on Oahu, specifically for registered nurse students. As VP, she began the process with 18 students, and over the next 14 years, she developed and implemented undergraduate and graduate degree programs to grow the student body to approximately 900 students. Programs included business, practical nurse to RN, RN to BSN, family nurse practitioner, mental health counseling, teacher special education and others. During these years, she also opened a small private practice for the management of sexual issues.

Her overall nursing experiences include medical-surgical, intensive care, rehabilitation, AIDS and HIV, nurse administration, nurse education, business education, human sexuality, obstetrics, and rehabilitation.

Credentials include a RN to BSN, MSN, MBA, and a PhD in Human Sexuality.

Awards include the Sigma Theta Tau Excellence in Nursing Award (1989); The American Organization of Nurse Executives Nurse Executive of the Year Award, Hawaii (2005); The Utah Governor's Humanitarian Award for service to people with AIDS (1989); Governor Linda Lingle declared September 19th Grace Blodgett Day in Hawaii for her service to nursing and education (2005).

Visit Dr. Gracie online at:

www.UnderstandingPatientsSexualProblems.com

NOTES: